"Written with moving clarity and deep compassion, this book brings together psychoanalytic insight and evidence-based practice in a truly integrative way, widening the frame beyond protocol and offering clinicians a framework for listening beneath symptoms to the emotional storms endured by adolescents living with OCD. This book manages a rare achievement of being both conceptually robust and pragmatically adaptable."

Dr Rosa Hoshi, *MSc, PhD, DClinPsy, C. Psychol, HCPC Reg Senior Tutor & Equality Diversity, Lead, Chartered Clinical Psychologist, Cardiff University*

"This is a rare and remarkable book, that blends clinical insight with genuine heartfelt dedication to young people struggling with OCD. Clinicians will find practical guidance, rich psychological nuances and the writers compassionate voice that strengthens both their understanding and therapeutic presence."

Dr Manisha Kale, *PhD, C.Psychol, HCPC Reg, UKCP (Systemic Psychotherapist), Chartered Clinical Psychologist & Systemic Psychotherapist, Child and Adolescent Mental Health Services (CAMHS)*

"As a psychotherapist working with families of distressed adolescents, I found this book a refreshingly clear summary of key ideas and concepts for clinicians at all stages working with OCD specifically, and with adolescence more generally."

Dr Anthony Brown, *C.Psychol AFBPsS, Specialist Family & Systemic Psychotherapist, Child and Adolescent Mental Health Services (CAMHS)*

"This book is an invaluable resource rich, insightful, and deeply stimulating. Working daily with young people who experience obsessive-like symptoms, I found its practical strategies and fresh perspectives transformative."

Megan Squire *BSc (Hons), MSc Health Psychology, Child and Adolescent Mental Health Support Worker, CAMHS*

"I am delighted to recommend this timely book, which addresses a topic that is both bewildering and fascinating for clinicians. As Dr Lewton's book rightly highlights, a sizeable proportion of cases involving children and young people with OCD know intellectually that compulsions do not reduce their exposure to harm."

Dr Misbah Gladwyn-Khan, *DClinPsy, C.Psychol, HCPC Reg (Clinical Psychologist) Adult Mental Health Services*

Intrusive Thoughts and Compulsions in Adolescent OCD

This comprehensive and clinically focused volume offers a therapeutic framework for understanding and treating intrusive thoughts and compulsions in adolescents with obsessive-compulsive disorder (OCD). By bridging theory and practice, it provides clinicians with the tools to explore the emotional and symbolic dimensions of OCD, fostering deeper therapeutic engagement.

Grounded in post-Kleinian and Bionian theory, the book offers a structural reading of obsessive-compulsive symptoms, shifting focus from surface content to the psychic architecture beneath. Through vivid clinical vignettes, annotated transcripts and practical interventions, Marcus Lewton equips clinicians with the skills to recognise and address the unique emotional stances adolescents take toward their OCD symptoms. The book integrates psychoanalytic insights with structured cross-modal approaches such as exposure response prevention (ERP) and cognitive behavioural therapy (CBT), emphasising patience, attunement and the symbolic meaning behind compulsions. Alongside detailed clinical material, the book provides guidance on tracking emotional and relational movement in therapy, communicating with parents and working thoughtfully with complex dynamics in adolescent treatment.

This book is ideal for clinicians across disciplines – from psychologists and psychiatrists to social workers and educators – working with adolescents experiencing OCD. It is a valuable resource for advanced students and researchers in child and adolescent mental health, offering a nuanced perspective that combines psychoanalytic depth with evidence-based practices.

Marcus Lewton is a child and adolescent clinical psychologist based in the UK. His work in independent practice and public services focuses on a wide range of adolescent mental health issues, with a specialist interest in intrusive thoughts and OCD.

Intrusive Thoughts and Compulsions in Adolescent OCD

A Psychoanalytic Framework for Treatment

Marcus Lewton

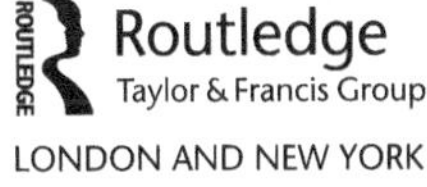

Routledge
Taylor & Francis Group

LONDON AND NEW YORK

Designed cover image: © Getty Images

First published 2026
by Routledge
4 Park Square, Milton Park, Abingdon, Oxon OX14 4RN

and by Routledge
605 Third Avenue, New York, NY 10158

Routledge is an imprint of the Taylor & Francis Group, an informa business

© 2026 Marcus Lewton

For Product Safety Concerns and Information please contact our EU representative GPSR@taylorandfrancis.com. Taylor & Francis Verlag GmbH, Kaufingerstraße 24, 80331 München, Germany.

British Library Cataloguing in Publication Data
A catalogue record for this book is available from the British Library

Library of Congress Cataloging-in-Publication Data
A catalog record has been requested for this book

ISBN: 978-1-041-21920-0 (hbk)
ISBN: 978-1-041-21919-4 (pbk)
ISBN: 978-1-003-72971-6 (ebk)

DOI: 10.4324/9781003729716

Typeset in Times New Roman
by Taylor & Francis Books

To every adolescent who has sat across from me and asked, 'What if this thought means I'm bad?' Your courage, honesty, and search for understanding inspired this book and reflect the hope that understanding brings. I also dedicate this work to the psychoanalytic thinkers, writers, supervisors, and colleagues who taught me to think analytically, imaginatively, and poetically. They showed me how to remain grounded in the room, even when helplessness, hopelessness, and uncertainty fill the air. From them I learned that simply being with another mind, instead of rushing to intervene, is often the most meaningful act. Finally, I dedicate this book to Dr Michelle Wells, an exceptional clinical psychologist who trained alongside me and tragically passed away. She was known in our cohort as the warmest, kindest trainee, deeply committed to marginalised groups. As the saying goes, she was 'beautiful inside and out'.

Contents

Boxes

Disclaimer

The views, opinions, and clinical models presented in this book are solely those of the author. They do not necessarily reflect the official stance, policy, or practices of any employer, including but not limited to the National Health Service (NHS) or affiliated organisations.

This work is for informational and educational purposes only. It does not replace formal clinical supervision, professional training, or personalised mental health care. Readers should seek expert advice for specific cases or concerns.

All case examples have been anonymised or fictionalised solely to ensure confidentiality. Any resemblance to actual persons, living or dead, is purely coincidental unless explicitly stated otherwise.

The author assumes no responsibility for errors, omissions, or outcomes resulting from the use of information contained herein. If you are struggling with your mental health, please seek help from a qualified professional.

Foreword

This book is not a manifesto. It is a clinical framework, a map that aligns with what many clinicians intuitively sense. Intrusive thoughts in adolescence are not mere cognitive noise. They land like signals from the mind's interior. Fear, guilt, shame, all bound up inside them. This is not a book of strict protocols. It is about the emotional stances young people take in relation to their intrusive thoughts and compulsions, how they cope, defend, and survive, and it calls clinicians to stand alongside them with attunement as well as technique.

I have written this for the clinicians who have delivered exposure and response prevention (ERP) as part of cognitive behavioural therapy (CBT), provided the right psychoeducation, asked the right questions, set up the right homework, and supported families in resisting accommodation, yet still find themselves sitting across from a young person whose gaze has become a kind of emotional absence. I have written it for those who engage, who persist, who do the work, and still feel quietly ambushed by the strangeness of their own mind. I have also written it with families in mind, those suspended in that tense space between compassion and confusion, watching someone they love disappear behind compulsions that make no sense yet will not let go, bringing immense suffering both to the young person and to the family system.

This book is not about replacing CBT, which includes ERP. Cognitive behavioural therapy, particularly when combined with ERP, continues to be the leading psychological treatment for obsessive-compulsive disorder (OCD), as outlined in guidance from the National Institute for Health and Care Excellence (NICE, 2005) and reaffirmed in NICE's most recent review at the time of writing (2024).

Yet even empirically driven protocols, supported by decades of research and outcome measures, have limits. Clinical presentations often defy strict categorisation, and many adolescents do not respond predictably to structured exposure exercises. Not every clinician finds clarity when symptoms are plainly debilitating. Sometimes the room is filled only with stillness and silence, with little therapeutic connection at all. This book is about widening the frame so that moments and presentations that fall outside protocol can still be recognised, held, and worked with.

I begin with a question: where is this young person, emotionally and internally, right now? Everything that follows is an attempt to sit with that question, think about it, and act from it.

This book is about stance, attention, and patience, about the discipline of staying in contact with the young person's inner world, even when that world feels unreachable. To work in this way is to notice how an adolescent relates to their intrusive thoughts and compulsions, and to respond not only with technique but with presence. It asks us to be clinicians who can tolerate not knowing, who can sit with ambiguity without rushing to resolve it, and who can wait long enough for something real to emerge.

The positions described here are not mine in origin. They belong to a lineage of theory and clinical thought that long predates me. My ambition has been to bring them off the page and into the rooms where young people are seen today. To do this, they must be translated, not diluted, into a language that can live in contemporary child and adolescent mental health practice without losing their force or originality.

I recognise that many qualified psychoanalysts may not fully endorse the approach I outline here, and I understand why. Psychoanalysis, taken in its unmodified form, is not merely a set of interventions but a way of living and thinking, cultivated through long immersion in a tradition that prizes depth, precision, and fidelity. There is an integrity to that purity, and I acknowledge the risk that any adaptation might be seen as compromise. Yet in the present climate of child and adolescent mental health, where pressures are relentless and the consequences of untreated distress can echo through a lifetime, I believe there is an ethical and therapeutic necessity to work with what we have, drawing upon the richness of the psychoanalytic canon while shaping it to meet contemporary clinical practice.

From the other side, colleagues trained in more manualised or protocol-driven approaches may question whether psychoanalytic ideas, often dismissed as outdated or opaque, have any place here. My view is that this perception, while not without cause, misreads the situation. Psychoanalytic theory offers profound and enduring insights, yet its challenge lies in translating these complex ideas into practical, accessible tools for contemporary clinical environments.

Adolescence sharpens this point. With puberty comes a surge of sexual and aggressive impulses, heightened moral awareness, and new capacities for abstract thought. Intrusive thoughts at this stage are not random. They clash with the turbulence of bodily change, emerging sexuality, and the adolescent's struggle to hold guilt, desire, and dread together. Compulsions often arise as desperate attempts to repair this collision, to restore certainty where development has made certainty impossible. If we fail to name this developmental storm, we risk mistaking its symptoms for simple resistance or non-engagement.

As a clinical psychologist, I stand partly within and partly beyond the psychoanalytic world. My training requires me to hold multiple psychological perspectives in mind, to test each critically, and to integrate where value is found. My commitment is to take what psychoanalysis offers in its richness and depth, its curiosity about unconscious life, and its concern with meaning, and make it workable in a setting where time is short, resources are stretched, and the young person's future is in the balance. This is not dilution. It is translation, so that psychoanalytic thought does not remain confined to the past but continues to illuminate and elevate the care we offer today.

If there is one hope that carries through these pages, it is this. We must try to keep hold of the human thread, even in the midst of method. Symptoms often emerge as adaptive responses to internal distress, and compulsions may serve as urgent strategies to preserve a sense of psychological coherence.

Acknowledgements

This book would not exist without the courage and trust of the young people and families who shared their experiences with me.

I also thank Dr Manisha Kale and Dr Tony Brown for accompanying me on this journey, for sharing their insights, and for tolerating the unpredictability of child and adolescent mental health services. I am equally grateful to Professor Brett Kahr, whose writing, podcasts, and unwavering advocacy for psychoanalysis inspired me to write.

Finally, to my family, whose laughter, nourishment, and love sustained me, and to my parents, who provided what Winnicott (1953) called a 'good enough' environment. Without them, this book would not exist.

References

National Institute for Health and Care Excellence (NICE). (2005; updated 2024). *Obsessive-compulsive disorder and body dysmorphic disorder: Treatment (Clinical guideline 31)*. London: NICE.

Winnicott, D. W. (1953). Transitional objects and transitional phenomena. *International Journal of Psycho-Analysis*, 34, 89–97.

A Note for Clinicians

This book is written for clinicians across behavioural, psychodynamic, systemic, and integrative traditions. Its aim is to deepen practice and sharpen clinical attention. Because work with young people always unfolds in a wider caregiving context, several of the main chapters include short sections titled Guidance for Parents (for clinicians to use when communicating with families). The title is kept for stylistic clarity, but these sections are intended more broadly. They can be used when working with parents, primary caregivers, or other systems around the adolescent. Their purpose is to equip clinicians with language that reduces shame, avoids jargon, and fosters steadiness at home and in the wider network. These are not parent-led materials but clinician-facing tools.

The framework presented here is deliberately flexible. Its focus is on what often remains unspoken in obsessive-compulsive disorder (OCD) presentations, particularly in adolescents whose intrusive thoughts or images carry moral weight or symbolic meaning. By symbolic meaning, I mean that the thoughts and even the compulsions do not always represent what their surface content suggests (for example, fear of germs or someone dying). They can stand in for other experiences, emotional conflicts, or feelings that have not yet been thought about or verbalised. What matters is less the literal content of the obsession and compulsion than the position the adolescent takes in relation to it.

Each of the four position chapters follows a consistent structure. Each begins with a conceptualisation of the position, outlining its emotional logic. Clinical examples and transcripts illustrate how the stance emerges in dialogue. Attention is then given to recognising its features in the consulting room, followed by interventions tailored in pacing, framing, and language. Short sections on communicating with parents or caregivers provide clinicians with family-facing language, and each chapter closes with a concise summary of key points.

This book is not a treatment manual but a way of listening beneath the surface of symptoms and fear. To listen in this way is to prioritise depth over certainty, process over protocol, and to remain close to the young person's lived experience, even when it resists neat formulation. Uncertainty, in this approach, is not a gap in technique but a necessary condition for therapeutic work.

Nowadays, services face rising demand and pressure for quick fixes and solutions to complex and evolving problems. This framework offers a way to think deeply while remaining clinically practical. Just as OCD seeks certainty through repetition, this book resists premature closure. It invites clinicians to linger in uncertainty, to notice the meanings intrusive thoughts and rituals conceal, and to hold open the space where new possibilities can emerge.

Although written as a clinical resource rather than an academic text, references are included where useful. They are offered not to burden the reader with scholarship, but to provide a bridge between practice and theory, grounding clinical intuition in established psychological thinking while keeping the book accessible, flexible, and alive in clinical practice.

A Note on Language

Throughout this book I use the word *clinician* rather than *therapist*. This is purposeful. Young people with intrusive thoughts and compulsive symptoms are encountered not only in psychology and psychiatry but also in nursing, social work, and education. My aim is that the ideas here are usable across disciplines, not confined to a single professional identity. Where clinical transcripts are included, I keep the label Therapist for clarity of dialogue, but the principles apply to any professional working with adolescents in distress.

Throughout the book I also use the terms adolescent and young person interchangeably. This is for stylistic variety, but, unless otherwise specified, each refers to the 12–18 years age group.

When writing about adolescents, I use he and she as pronouns for stylistic simplicity, while recognising the diverse ways young people experience and express gender. Adolescence is often a time of transition and exploration of identity, and the clinical principles described here apply equally to young people of all gender identities.

Cultural context also shapes the way intrusive thoughts and compulsions are experienced and spoken about. In some settings, they may be framed through religious or moral lenses; in others, through medical or familial ones. The language I use in this book is rooted in my own clinical practice, but the framework is intended to be adapted in dialogue with the cultural and faith traditions that shape the lives of young people and their families.

Chapter 1

The Heart of It

A 16-year-old sits in silence, convinced that a single thought has made her dangerous. She avoids knives, scissors, even pencils, terrified that even being near them might unleash violence. Her world grows smaller each week, while her parents watch helplessly, their faces carrying the same fear she cannot put into words.

I have watched parents cry, convinced their child might be turning into a monster. I have listened to families voice fears that their adolescent is 'going crazy', or that disturbing thoughts must be signs of perversion. Teachers and professionals too find themselves in panic, uncertain how to respond. I have sat with young people too afraid to speak their thoughts aloud, not even to themselves. I have received referrals from crisis teams in emergency departments, where adolescents have arrived with suicidal thoughts and plans, driven not by psychosis or severe depression but by the unbearable pressure of repetitive, terrifying intrusive thoughts.

Intrusive thoughts do not just unsettle. They haunt and they hunt. They take up space in an adolescent's mind, leaving little room for anything else. In doing so, they derail ordinary growth: progressing through education, developing friendships, experimenting with identities and ways of being. These are the very experiences that should be foundational at this stage. And, despite their weight, they are often dismissed, misunderstood, or met with hollow reassurance: 'Just ignore it. It's only a thought.' It rarely helps. Often, it makes it worse.

The wider culture, too, misreads these experiences. Again and again, intrusive thoughts are mistaken for intent or, more historically, for morbid repressed wishes. Both readings misjudge the phenomenon. What is private torment can so quickly become public catastrophe.

For adolescents, this misunderstanding is magnified. With puberty comes a surge of sexual and aggressive feelings, heightened moral awareness, and new capacities for abstract thought. As Meltzer and Harris (1986) observed from their decades of work with adolescents, this stage is not simply the arrival of new feelings, but a restructuring of the emotional architecture already laid down in infancy and childhood. Old anxieties resurface, now tested against

DOI: 10.4324/9781003729716-1

the demand to take up new roles, new responsibilities, and new forms of independence across both public and private settings. Yet the pull back to dependence remains just as powerful, creating a constant tension between clinging and breaking away. Intrusive thoughts enter this turbulence with force, conflicting not only with bodily change but also with the complexity of contemporary social worlds, both offline and online, where identities are scrutinised, exposed, and compared. Compulsions arise as desperate attempts to restore certainty and safety in the midst of this turbulent restructuring. What might once have been a passing childhood fear can, in adolescence, become a torment that feels both shaming and overwhelming.

The Reassurance Dilemma

In my clinical work, I have seen families unravel under panic, anxiety, and grief. I have met parents who ask, through tears and helplessness, whether their child could be a sex offender, a murderer, or a psychopath. They can't help but wonder if these intrusive thoughts are early warning signs that something is fundamentally wrong with their child's mind. 'Why on earth would she have those disgusting thoughts?' one anxious and distressed father asked me. I have seen adolescents obsessively checking their own minds, terrified that a thought might define who they are or predict who they will become.

As a clinician, one of the hardest instincts to resist is the urge to reassure. To say, 'You're fine. It's just a thought. Many adolescents get them. Don't worry, they mean nothing.' Sometimes that is exactly what the young person or parent longs to hear. But reassurance, while briefly soothing, is rarely transformative. At best, it offers a pause in the storm. At worst, it slides into the compulsive cycle itself. The adolescent begins to lean on the clinician's words for moral safety, as though reassurance alone could prove that they remain good, kind, or safe. Over time, reassurance risks becoming a ritual in its own right.

Reassurance may calm for a moment, but it flips the old adage of 'short-term pain for long-term gain'. Here, the short-term gain deepens the long-term pain. Families often grasp this in principle, yet when they are with their child at home or in public it becomes almost impossible to refrain. The distress an adolescent feels when reassurance is withheld can be unbearable for everyone in the room. Parents frequently tell me, 'I know I'm not helping but I cannot see him that distressed,' or, 'I know it doesn't help, but her worries stop immediately if I just do it for her. Otherwise she'll be up for hours and wrecked for school.' It is hard not to collude with this logic. Who can honestly say they would easily withstand their child's anguish and tolerate their own helplessness? Yet, if the adolescent is to be given a fighting chance, accommodation must be resisted.

Thoughts and Compulsions

While they are distinct, obsessions and compulsions cannot be separated. Some compulsions are visible and stereotypical, the ones that immediately come to mind when people think of obsessive-compulsive disorder (OCD): checking that doors are locked, washing hands, arranging objects symmetrically, tapping furniture a set number of times. Others are subtle, even hidden: silent prayers, repeated phrases, mental replays. Some involve touching the body, or particular breathing patterns. The variety is as endless as human behaviour itself.

Technology now plays a striking role in these subtler compulsions. Many adolescents have told me they must open certain apps a set number of times or scroll through reels for a specific duration before they feel safe. These compulsions are not evolving so much as adapting to modern conditions.

Whatever their form, the function is the same: to neutralise or undo the thought, to ward off an imagined catastrophe. Intrusive thoughts in adolescence must always be understood together with the compulsions that accompany them. Clinicians can sometimes become preoccupied with the rituals themselves, cataloguing each sequence in detail, in the hope that precision will unlock meaning. This is usually a red herring. The form matters less than the function. Compulsions are attempts to relieve the anguish a thought provokes. Staying with that distress is what is key.

What truly drives the anxiety is not the thought itself but the meaning the adolescent assigns to it. How they interpret and make sense of the thought shapes the urge to neutralise. This can be extraordinarily difficult to accept when the thought feels alien, entirely at odds with the kind of person they know themselves to be.

Adolescence makes this pairing especially powerful. The same imagination that once led a child to believe they could heal a sore knee by touching it or saying a magic word may now fuel the conviction that a thought alone could cause harm. What was once playful or adaptive in early childhood returns as torment, bringing psychological distress and disruption across schooling, friendships, social life, and identity.

Listening Differently

What I do instead is listen actively, with precision and curiosity, resisting assumptions even when a case feels familiar or I feel I've heard the story for the umpteenth time. As Wilfred Bion, a leading figure in psychoanalysis, suggested, genuine understanding requires the suspension of memory and desire (Bion, 1970). If I enter the room expecting to recognise the story, I risk flattening its nuance. If I empathise too quickly, I risk imposing my own meanings on the adolescent's pain, making assumptions before the young mind in front of me has had the chance to share their story in their own way.

This is not always easy. Public services are often commissioned for a set number of sessions, with external pressures to formulate quickly and move toward behavioural interventions. Line managers, senior teams, and service directors are tasked with ensuring equity and effectiveness. We cannot overhaul policy or see adolescents indefinitely, but within limits we can still hold on to the importance of listening. Even brief contact allows for listening that is careful and humane.

To work well with intrusive thoughts and compulsions, I must approach each young person with openness. That means attending not only to what is spoken, but to tone, silences, avoided subjects. It means noticing what the adolescent evokes in me and asking what that might reveal. It requires presence, patience, and a willingness to stay near the internal world behind the words. One might argue that this stance is the hallmark of all good clinicians, yet when faced with something as overt and pressing as OCD, the skill of listening can easily be lost.

Same Symptom, Different Worlds

I once worked with two adolescents, both of whom met diagnostic criteria for OCD and scored similarly on well-validated measures of severity. On paper, they were indistinguishable. They came from similar socioeconomic backgrounds, and their family systems looked much the same. Yet, in the room, symptom and psyche were interwoven in radically different ways.

Both were tormented by the same thought: what if I stab my little sister? Both carried out compulsions to check that the environment was safe. Both avoided being left alone with their sister. Both sought reassurance from parents that they would never harm her. On paper, the content of the thought and the behaviour was identical. In practice, they were worlds apart.

One boy avoided my gaze, speaking quickly and defensively. He insisted he did not care, yet circled back again and again to whether I thought he was 'messed up'. The room felt tight, as though I were being tested. For him, the thought arrived as an intrusion, violent and persecutory. He was under siege and managed his distress with fleeting minimisation before turning to me for reassurance.

The other boy whispered the same thought with tears in his eyes, convinced it revealed something irredeemable about his soul. He spoke of his sister with warmth but feared he might destroy her, not out of hatred but because his love felt dangerous. His relation to the thought was saturated with grief and guilt.

The symptoms were identical. The psychic positions they occupied in relation to those symptoms could not have been more different.

These two boys remind me why checklists and symptom measures, useful as they are, can never capture the whole picture. Symptom counts tell us what the adolescent is doing, but not what the act means to them. Without listening for the psychic position, we risk treating every compulsion as though it were the same, when in fact the same ritual may arise from entirely different anxieties and emotional configurations. One boy defended against intrusion with denial and sought reassurance as a shield against persecution. The other collapsed into guilt, as if his very capacity for love marked him as dangerous. To treat them as identical cases because their forms of OCD looked the same would be to miss the point altogether.

Beyond Symptoms: Psychic Positions

When I use the word psychic, I do not mean mysticism or clairvoyance. I mean it in the psychoanalytic sense: the inner world every mind inhabits, often unspoken but deeply felt. Each person has a psychic architecture, an internal scaffolding of development and defence beneath outward behaviour and personality. This scaffolding is laid down in infancy, shaped by temperament, genetics, and the first relationships that hold, or fail to hold, the child. In the years of middle childhood, roughly 6 to 11, it is built upon by curiosity, a growing social world, and the acquisition of skills and knowledge. In adolescence, this architecture is tested, stretched, sometimes destabilised, when intrusive thoughts and compulsions collide with new sexual feelings, a developing moral compass, heightened emotional reactivity, and the task of forming an identity.

Early in my career, I tried to organise presentations of OCD in adolescence by themes: contamination, violence, blasphemy, sexuality. I applied rating scales and psychometric measures of severity. Yet the symptoms repeated themselves more in form than in meaning, and the numbers could not explain why two adolescents with identical scores felt so utterly different in the room. I discovered that, while useful as a starting point, this way of categorising did not deepen my understanding.

Over time, I began to notice something else. Beneath the surface themes, young people seemed to adopt recognisable stances in relation to their intrusive thoughts and compulsions. These were not diagnostic subtypes, but what I came to see as psychic positions – specific ways of relating to their thoughts, their compulsions, and to me.

These positions were not new. Psychoanalytic literature had described them long before my training, even before my birth: the claustrum (Meltzer, 1992), the paranoid–schizoid and depressive positions (Klein, 1940, 1946), and the psychic retreat (Steiner, 1993). These ideas had not been applied directly to adolescents with OCD, yet they illuminated what I encountered daily. In the claustrum, inquiry about compulsions or intrusive thoughts was met with impenetrable silence, the atmosphere not merely stuck but trapped. In the paranoid–schizoid position, compulsions were driven by projections of danger, the fear that catastrophe would strike them or their loved ones if the ritual was not performed. In the psychic retreat, symptoms waxed and waned: one week minimal, the next overwhelming, as the adolescent disappeared into OCD to keep conflict at bay. In the depressive position, the young person wanted to challenge compulsions and make peace with their thoughts, but was weighed down by grief, guilt, and loss.

The Central Claim

Through reflection and supervision, four positions became central to my clinical practice:

- The claustrum, where the adolescent walls off from emotional contact.
- The paranoid–schizoid position, where danger is projected outward.
- The psychic retreat, where functioning continues but with inner withdrawal.
- The depressive position, where guilt, self-blame, and emotional honesty come to the fore.

Each demands a different therapeutic stance. Some adolescents need containment. Others need challenge. Some can tolerate exposure. Others cannot.

This book offers a framework not only for what to treat, but for who we meet in the process. Its central claim is simple: intrusive thoughts and compulsions in adolescence are best understood through psychic position. When we can see where a young person is standing internally, we can begin to offer them a way forward, a way out.

Roadmap of the Book

Having introduced the core claim, the chapters ahead walk through each position in detail, offering clinical examples, therapeutic strategies, and reflections from the consulting room.

I begin with Chapter 2, which examines how OCD is typically conceptualised and categorised in everyday clinical practice. It highlights the limits of categorical diagnosis and points of overlap with other conditions such as autism.

Chapter 3 adopts a developmental lens, tracing how ordinary experiences from infancy can resurface in adolescence as intrusive thoughts and compulsions. It explores key mechanisms such as omnipotence, splitting, and an inflated sense of responsibility, using clinical examples to show how these processes parallel the presentations we encounter in the consulting room.

In Chapter 4, I explore the turbulence of adolescent development itself, showing how sexuality, morality, and identity struggles inflame the residues described in Chapter 3. This provides a developmental arc that connects early experiences to adolescent life, and explains why adolescence is the stage when intrusive thoughts and compulsions so often intensify.

Chapter 5 offers a selective review of wider psychoanalytic ideas that inform the current framework, showing how meaning and affect shape intrusive thoughts and rituals. It highlights how intrusive phenomena are often linked to deeper, unexpressed feelings and experiences.

Reflecting on the current clinical climate, Chapter 6 reviews the evidence base for OCD treatment in adolescence, noting what the data shows is effective and where its limits lie. It also considers the mechanisms underlying exposure and response prevention, and how these are applied in treatment.

Chapter 7 provides an orienting bridge into the position chapters. It outlines how to discern stance in the room and how this shapes intervention. It explains the common structure of the position chapters: defining the concept through clinical examples, presenting therapy transcripts, examining how the position appears in the room, and offering guidance on clinical work, including communication with primary caregivers.

Chapter 8 opens with the claustrum, a position in which the adolescent walls off from emotional contact. It discusses the challenges that arise when working with such a closed-down state of mind.

In Chapter 9, I turn to the Psychic Retreat, where an adolescent may appear to be improving and functioning well, with OCD symptoms fading almost overnight, only for them to return with full intensity when emotional experience is stirred. This chapter explores the function of this position and ways of working with it clinically.

Chapter 10 considers the paranoid–schizoid position, a well-established concept in psychoanalysis. Here, danger is projected outward and splitting predominates. The chapter highlights the challenges of working with such a persecutory state of mind.

The position chapters conclude with Chapter 11, which explores the depressive position, where guilt, self-blame, and emotional honesty come to the fore, creating the possibility of reparation.

Chapter 12 reflects on how research might evolve to capture and measure these processes, while also recognising the challenge of studying what is often invisible in the room. It considers how research methods have changed, the limits of existing approaches, and the importance of teaching clinicians to remain attuned to the clinical texture of sessions.

Finally, Chapter 13 offers a brief reflective essay, drawing the book together and anticipating the current challenges and future directions in work with adolescents with OCD.

Before we descend into those depths, however, we must pause at the surface to examine how OCD is usually conceptualised, and why intrusive thoughts and compulsions so often slip through the cracks. Only then can we begin to see the architecture beneath.

References

Bion, W. R. (1970). *Attention and interpretation: A scientific approach to insight in psycho-analysis and groups.* London: Tavistock Publications.

Klein, M. (1940). Mourning and its relation to manic-depressive states. *International Journal of Psycho-Analysis*, 21, 125–153.

Klein, M. (1946). Notes on some schizoid mechanisms. *International Journal of Psycho-Analysis*, 27, 99–110.

Meltzer, D. (1992). *The claustrum: An investigation of claustrophobic phenomena.* Perthshire: Clunie Press.

Meltzer, D., & Harris, M. (1986). *Adolescence: Talks and papers.* Perthshire: Clunie Press.

Steiner, J. (1993). *Psychic retreats: Pathological organizations in psychotic, neurotic and borderline patients.* London: Routledge.

Chapter 2

Beyond the Label

Differentiating OCD in Practice

In this chapter I turn to how obsessive-compulsive disorder (OCD) is typically defined and conceptualised in contemporary clinical practice. Diagnostic manuals and research papers list causes and categories, but in the consulting room they arrive as lived experience: an adolescent who panics that he might become like his father; a girl convinced her rituals mean she is following her mother's path; a family struggling to make sense of a sudden onset that has negatively impacted the entire family system. To understand OCD in adolescence we must hold these fragments together without mistaking them for the whole story.

Conceptual Maps

Too often, OCD is spoken of as if it were a single fixed disorder, a neatly bordered category into which certain thoughts and behaviours fall. Many clinicians, myself included, and many parents might wish this were so. It would allow us to apply a specific intervention and expect steady symptom relief, a straightforward improvement in quality of life. But clinical reality rarely grants us that simplicity.

In practice, OCD is less like a single map and more like navigating backstreets in an old cathedral city. You turn down a lane you think you know, only to find it bends back on itself. A steep flight of steps may look familiar, yet from another angle feel entirely new. In the consulting room, what first appears a familiar symptom often reveals a different logic when explored from a fresh perspective. Both the young person and the clinician can feel briefly disoriented, searching for bearings.

The *Diagnostic and Statistical Manual of Mental Disorders, Fifth Edition* (DSM-5; APA, 2013) and the *International Classification of Diseases, Eleventh Revision* (ICD-11; WHO, 2019) define OCD in terms of obsessions, unwanted intrusive thoughts, images or urges, and compulsions, the repetitive behaviours or mental acts performed to reduce distress or prevent catastrophe. There must be a direct link between the compulsion and the obsession. For example, a young person with OCD must be able to link an

DOI: 10.4324/9781003729716-2

intrusive thought with carrying out a specific compulsion. For a formal diagnosis, these compulsions typically take up a significant amount of time, often an hour or more each day, and interfere with ordinary life. In adolescence, the cost is conspicuous in school, friendships, family relationships, and general wellbeing. I often hear adolescents protest they are not lazy. The moment they try to begin the day, they are hit by an onslaught of rituals and thoughts so relentless that staying in bed feels less unbearable. These thoughts are typically described as ego-dystonic, meaning experienced as alien to who they are. A kind boy tormented by violent images. A devout girl plagued by blasphemous ideas. By contrast, ego-syntonic traits, those felt as part of the self, provoke far less torment.

Intrusive thoughts are sometimes described more broadly as obsessions, and they can also appear in trauma, depression, or other conditions. Here, my focus is specifically on intrusive thoughts in OCD, because in this disorder they almost always come bound to compulsions that attempt to undo or contain them. It is precisely this pairing that sets OCD apart, making the experience more consuming and qualitatively different from other presentations in which intrusive thoughts may occur.

Another requirement for diagnosis is that the clinical presentation cannot better be explained by another disorder such as substance misuse, a tic disorder, or body dysmorphia. Beyond these criteria, a holistic assessment should include a clinical interview with the adolescent, informant reports from parents, teachers, siblings, or significant others, and administration of a validated measure such as the Children's Yale–Brown Obsessive Compulsive Scale (CY-BOCS) (Scahill et al., 1997) or its updated version, the CY-BOCS-II (Storch et al., 2019).

For many clinicians and families, the DSM and ICD criteria offer a relieving starting point. A formal diagnosis can bring a measure of peace of mind. It gives parents and young people a name for what is happening and a shared language for colleagues and services. Schools and colleges often become more accommodating where before they might have taken a stricter approach. Yet these labels remain limited. They rarely illuminate the subjective experience of OCD, what it feels like to carry the fear, how a compulsion functions in the moment, or what it means for the adolescent's inner world.

The *Psychodynamic Diagnostic Manual, Second Edition* (PDM-2; Lingiardi & McWilliams, 2017) offers something different. It describes not only symptoms but inner life: how a person manages emotion, the conflicts beneath difficulties, and the stance they take toward themselves and others. To me, this feels closer to the reality of the young people I meet. Yet it remains outside the mainstream. Unlike DSM or ICD, the PDM-2 is rarely used in everyday services or commissioning frameworks, limiting its visibility and influence. This is striking because it provides insights that can deepen our understanding of adolescents with OCD and help bridge the gap between symptoms and lived experience.

In practice, one of the clearest ways I have found to hold this gap is by distinguishing between situational and structural presentations of OCD.

Situational and Structural OCD

In clinical work, I often distinguish between what I call *situational* OCD and *structural* OCD. These are not formal subtypes listed in any diagnostic manual, but I have found the distinction clinically useful because it allows me to gauge how entrenched a presentation may be. It highlights important differences in depth, function, and therapeutic response.

In situational OCD, intrusive thoughts and compulsions arise in response to current stressors such as exam periods, relationship breakdowns, or sudden changes in circumstance. Symptoms are distressing, but when the stressor eases, they often settle predictably with standard treatment. This pattern is supported by research. While not specific to children or adolescence, a Japanese cohort study found that adults with OCD reported a recognisable stressor preceding onset (Murayama et al., 2020). Case reports, though anecdotal, show similar, whereby compulsions that emerge after bereavement, a frightening medical event, or even overhearing a traumatic story often improve rapidly with exposure and response prevention (ERP), sometimes within only a handful of sessions (Subramanian & Mayur, 2018).

Contemporary findings also align with what many clinicians observe. Stiede, Spencer, and Onyeka (2024) showed that early intervention for paediatric OCD is linked to improved psychological wellbeing. McGuire et al. (2015) reported that access to ERP and cognitive behavioural therapy (CBT) increased the likelihood of remission, even if some residual symptoms remained. A recent meta-analysis by Steele et al. (2025) concluded that combining ERP with medication offers significant benefit, particularly in more severe cases.

In my own practice, I see much the same. Adolescents seen soon after a stressor tend to improve faster. Anecdotally, in private practice, when young people can pinpoint a stressor, such as a breakup, and connect it to the onset of their OCD, they often respond more readily to a standardised approach. Of course, other factors may also play a role, but these patterns make intuitive sense to me.

I think of a girl whose checking rituals began after moving to a new school. She repeatedly opened her bag at the door to check her homework had not 'disappeared'. As school pressures eased, the checking reduced with standard ERP. She later said the ritual was 'the only way I could stop the panic', a reminder that even situational compulsions can feel overwhelming. Another boy, deeply attached to his friendship group, developed tapping rituals when quarrels erupted, fearing the group might split and leave him alone. Once the tensions passed, the compulsions subsided.

Structural OCD, by contrast, feels different for both adolescent and clinician. Symptoms may be triggered by a situation or stressor, but usually there is a longer developmental history, often reaching back into childhood. As the narrative unfolds, adolescents may recall early rituals or routines that once offered comfort. These patterns, dismissed at the time as harmless or 'just something I liked to do', later resurface with greater intensity.

What makes these behaviours structural is not only their persistence but the deeper meanings they take on. A door check may begin as a way of keeping the house safe but evolve into a way of holding the self together, locking away feelings of anger or negativity. A washing ritual may be less about germs than about cleansing guilt, shame, or rage. In this sense, compulsions shift from concrete acts to symbolic acts: checking a door to keep out burglars becomes checking to keep unbearable feelings from breaking through.

For readers more familiar with CBT or non-analytic approaches, it may feel like an imaginative leap to suggest that compulsions carry symbolic meaning. One might reasonably ask, where is the evidence? I will come back to this more fully in Chapter 6, but even without a psychoanalytic lens it is hard to ignore how compulsions evolve. They rarely stay neatly tied to the original fear. Over time, they stretch, mutate, take on new functions. This is not only my impression from clinical sessions with adolescents with OCD; longitudinal studies have also shown that symptom patterns do shift, sometimes quite markedly, even when the overall picture of OCD remains stable (Besiroglu et al., 2007; Obisie-Orlu et al., 2025). Put simply, the form may change, but the underlying struggle continues. This is why I am wary of taking compulsions at face value. They often grow into something larger than the thing they were first meant to ward off.

This symbolic layer is rarely conscious. It usually emerges only within the safety of a therapeutic relationship, where time and trust allow thoughts and feelings to surface. If one were to offer such interpretations too early, the adolescent would likely look perplexed, or simply not return.

Research supports this longer view. Longitudinal studies, that is, research studies that follow the same group of participants over time to see how their symptoms change, show that early-onset OCD often continues into later years (Geller et al., 2001; Micali et al., 2010). Register-based studies, which use national health or education records, add another layer of understanding. These studies (Pérez-Vigil et al., 2018, 2019) show that children diagnosed early with OCD are more likely to experience other mental health problems as they grow up and may find school or work more difficult.

These are the kinds of studies I think about when parents ask whether their child might just grow out of their OCD or whether it could be a phase. Sometimes that does happen, but these research findings remind us that OCD can leave deep and lasting marks if it is left unaddressed. It is one reason I believe early psychological help matters so much. The sooner we intervene, the better chance a young person has of finding relief and building a life that is not shaped by the illness.

In my experience, young people with structural presentations describe long histories of ritualised coping. Recognising this helps me pace the work carefully. I am transparent with parents and adolescents: behaviours relied upon for years to manage inner distress rarely vanish in a handful of sessions, however skilled or time-limited the intervention.

Distinguishing between situational and structural OCD is not about new categories; it is about stance. Situational cases often respond to exposure once stressors ease. Structural cases require slower work, building trust and attending to meaning before rituals can safely loosen. In structural presentations, compulsions have often become carriers of meaning, and the task is not simply to strip them away but to create conditions where their work is no longer needed.

Taken together, situational presentations usually arise in the context of identifiable stressors and, as research and practice both suggest, tend to remit more readily once those stressors resolve. Structural presentations by contrast often call for longer, relationship-centred work, helping the young person find words for what the rituals have been carrying.

Neurodiversity and OCD

Many autistic young people also meet criteria for OCD, yet the overlap can be a minefield to navigate. Rates vary, but meta-analytic estimates suggest that between 17 per cent and 37 per cent of autistic individuals meet criteria for OCD (van Steensel, Bögels, & Perrin, 2011). Repetitive behaviours, considered a hallmark feature of autism spectrum disorder (ASD), may appear identical to compulsions, but their underlying purpose is often phenomenologically different. A hand flap, a rocking movement, or an echo of words may soothe sensory overload rather than ward off catastrophe. The same gesture that regulates sensation in one child may, in another, be a ritual of safety. This is where the challenge lies: careful attention is needed to distinguish what appears to be a compulsion from what is, in fact, a way of regulating the self.

I recall an autistic adolescent who arranged his pencils into perfect lines before starting work. For him, this brought sensory calm. Another young person, also autistic, lined up pencils because she feared that if she did not, her family would die in the night. Outwardly the same action, inwardly worlds apart. What is imperative to remember is that compulsions are repetitive, but not all repetitive behaviours are compulsions. The overlap in form can mislead us, yet the underlying motivation is different: in autism, repetitive behaviours often regulate sensory or emotional states (van Steensel et al., 2011; Wu, Rudy, & Storch, 2014); while, in OCD, they almost always respond to an intrusive thought or fear (Aymerich et al., 2024; Dell'Osso et al., 2024).

I often find myself gently pointing out to colleagues that repetitive behaviours should not be too quickly dismissed as 'just autism', nor should sensory behaviours be mistakenly targeted with OCD protocols. Both misread the lived reality and risk leaving the adolescent unseen. The task is not to decide between labels but to listen carefully to how the young person themself understands what they do.

PANS and Sudden-Onset OCD

Some young people present not with a slow accumulation of rituals but with a sudden storm. A child who seemed settled on Monday may, by Wednesday, be unable to eat, sleep, or leave the house without repeating elaborate sequences. Parents describe it as if their son or daughter had been taken overnight.

This clinical picture has been called Paediatric Acute-onset Neuropsychiatric Syndrome (PANS), and, when linked to streptococcal infection, PANDAS. Research suggests that inflammatory or immune processes may play a role in the onset of this presentation, but the evidence remains mixed and widely debated (Johnson et al., 2019; Prato et al., 2021). For families, the experience is one of disorientation and loss, whether or not a precise medical cause is agreed.

I remember one mother who said: 'It was like he had been replaced in the night with someone else.' Another adolescent told me she woke one morning and felt her mind flood with fears she could not stop, as if a switch had been flipped.

Even here, where biology may dominate, the young person still occupies a psychic position in relation to their thoughts. Some feel besieged, others collapse into guilt as if the sudden change proves an inner corruption. Whatever the medical course, the symbolic stance remains part of the work.

Cultural and Social Media Influences

Today, many adolescents encounter OCD not first in a clinic but on TikTok, Instagram, or YouTube. They come having watched countless short videos about 'quirky' habits, often framed as light entertainment or identity. For some, this brings relief, a sense that they are not alone. For others, it deepens isolation, because the online version of OCD looks nothing like the torment they are living.

One 15-year-old girl described spending hours managing intrusive violent thoughts about her mother. When she confided in friends, they replied, 'I have OCD too, I hate it when my room is messy.' She fell silent, convinced no one could understand her reality. There is a deep cultural underestimation of how debilitating OCD can be. While social media can help normalise distress and remind people they are not alone, it can just as easily invalidate.

Research has echoed this. Analyses of TikTok content tagged #OCD often show the condition trivialised, portrayed as neatness or fussiness rather than distress (Woods & Gantt-Howrey, 2023). Broader reviews have confirmed that psychiatric disorders are particularly prone to false representation online (Fitzpatrick et al., 2025).

In my own practice, I often find myself balancing how I talk about this. It helps to reassure young people that intrusive thoughts are part of ordinary life, but if I lean too far in that direction they may feel I am minimising their suffering. Social media makes this balance more precarious; it spreads the term 'OCD' widely, but often in ways that erase its seriousness.

OCD and Obsessive Personality Organisation

In practice, one of the most common confusions is between OCD and obsessive personality traits. Parents, teachers, and even clinicians sometimes mistake a child's perfectionism for OCD, or dismiss compulsions as 'just personality'.

In OCD, the young person experiences thoughts and rituals as alien, unwanted, and distressing. A girl may scrub her hands until they bleed, desperate to rid herself of contamination, while insisting she hates the ritual. This is ego-dystonic suffering. By contrast, an adolescent with an obsessive personality organisation may spend hours perfecting homework, convinced it must be flawless. The behaviour may cause exhaustion or conflict, but it feels consistent with who they are.

Salzman's Obsessional Styles (1980) and McWilliams (2011) both make clear that these are different psychic structures, even if they sometimes overlap. In adolescence, the picture blurs further, as traits are still forming and the self is fluid. Premature personality labelling is best avoided (Sharp & Wall, 2018). What matters is to notice what the behaviour means. Is it an attempt to neutralise catastrophic fear or an expression of an inner law demanding control?

Conclusion

Looking across these perspectives, from diagnostic manuals to situational and structural distinctions, from neurodiversity to cultural influences, I am struck by how different each adolescent's story feels. Even when the symptoms look familiar on paper, the lived reality rarely repeats itself.

For adolescents, this struggle is sharpened by development itself. Puberty, sexuality, and moral awareness intensify the sense that thoughts may be dangerous and that rituals may be the only defence. Our task as clinicians is not simply to catalogue symptoms or trace causes, but to hear the stance each adolescent takes toward their own mind. That stance often tells us more than the symptom list.

The next chapter turns back to infancy, to the earliest psychic mechanisms that quietly persist into adolescence. Omnipotence, responsibility, splitting, and repetition begin as ordinary parts of survival. Later, they can resurface in distorted form, shaping the intrusive thoughts and compulsions that bring young people into the consulting room. To make sense of the adolescent mind, we have to understand these echoes of earliest life.

References

American Psychiatric Association (APA). (2013). *Diagnostic and statistical manual of mental disorders* (5th ed.). Arlington, VA: American Psychiatric Publishing. doi:10.1176/appi.books.9780890425596.

Aymerich, C., Pacho, M., Catalan, A., Yousaf, N., Pérez-Rodríguez, V., Hollocks, M. J., Parellada, M., Krebs, G., Clark, B., & Salazar de Pablo, G. (2024). Prevalence and correlates of the concurrence of autism spectrum disorder and obsessive compulsive disorder in children and adolescents: A systematic review and meta-analysis. *Brain Sciences*, 14(4), article 379. doi:10.3390/brainsci14040379.

Besiroglu, L., Uguz, F., Ozbebit, Ö., Güler, Ö., Çilli, A. S., & Askin, R. (2007). Longitudinal assessment of symptom and subtype categories in obsessive–compulsive disorder. *Depression and Anxiety*, 24(7), 461–466. doi:10.1002/da.20240.

Dell'Osso, L., Nardi, B., Bonelli, C., Amatori, G., Pereyra, M. A., Massimetti, E., Cremone, I. M., Pini, S., & Carpita, B. (2024). Autistic traits as predictors of increased obsessive–compulsive disorder severity: The role of inflexibility and communication impairment. *Brain Sciences*, 14(1), article 64. doi:10.3390/brainsci14010064.

Fitzpatrick, M., Moore, A. S., Kichuk, S. A., Pittenger, C., & Zaboski, B. A. (2025). #OCD: A content analysis of obsessive-compulsive disorder stereotype amplification and misinformation on TikTok. *Cyberpsychology, Behavior, and Social Networking*, 28(9), doi:10.1177/21522715251370135.

Geller, D. A., Biederman, J., Faraone, S. V., Bellordre, C. A., Kim, G. S., Hagermoser, L., Cradock, K., & Frazier, J. A. (2001). Developmental aspects of obsessive-compulsive disorder: Findings in children, adolescents, and adults. *The Journal of Nervous and Mental Disease*, 189(7), 471–477. doi:10.1097/00005053-200107000-00009.

Johnson, M., Fernell, E., Preda, I., Wallin, L., Fasth, A., Gilberg, C., & Gilberg, C. (2019). Paediatric acute-onset neuropsychiatric syndrome in children and adolescents: An observational cohort study. *The Lancet Child & Adolescent Health*, 3(8), 175–180. doi:10.1016/S2352-4642(18)30404-30408.

Lingiardi, V., & McWilliams, N. (Eds.). (2017). *Psychodynamic diagnostic manual: PDM-2*. New York: Guilford Press.

McGuire, J. F., Piacentini, J., Lewin, A. B., Brennan, E. A., Murphy, T. K., & Storch, E. A. (2015). A meta-analysis of cognitive behavior therapy and medication for child obsessive–compulsive disorder: Moderators of treatment efficacy, response, and remission. *Depression and Anxiety*, 32 (8), 580–593. doi:10.1002/da.22389.

McWilliams, N. (2011). *Psychoanalytic diagnosis: Understanding personality structure in the clinical process* (2nd ed.). New York: Guilford Press.

Micali, N., Heyman, I., Pérez, M., & Hilton, K. (2010). Long-term outcomes of obsessive–compulsive disorder: Follow-up of 142 children and adolescents. *The British Journal of Psychiatry*, 197(2), 128–134. doi:10.1192/bjp.bp.109.075317.

Murayama, K., Nakao, T., Ohno, A., Tsuruta, S., Tomiyama, H., Hasuzawa, S., Mizobe, T., Kato, K., & Kanba, S. (2020). Impacts of stressful life events and traumatic experiences on onset of obsessive-compulsive disorder. *Frontiers in Psychiatry*, 11, 561266. doi:10.3389/fpsyt.2020.561266.

Obisie-Orlu, I. C., Eisen, J. L., Rasmussen, S. A., & Boisseau, C. L. (2025). Stability and transition likelihood of primary symptoms in adults with obsessive-compulsive disorder: A 5-year prospective follow-up study. *Journal of Affect Disorders*, 381, 108–114, doi:10.1016/j.jad.2025.04.011.

Pérez-Vigil, A., Fernández de la Cruz, L., Brander, G., Isomura, K., Jangmo, A., Feldman, I., Hesselmark, E., Serlachius, E., Lázaro, L., Rück, C., Kuja-Halkola, R., D'Onofrio, B. M., Larsson, H., & Mataix-Cols, D. (2018). Association of obsessive-compulsive disorder with objective indicators of educational attainment: A nationwide register-based sibling control study. *JAMA Psychiatry*, 75(1), 47–55. doi:10.1001/jamapsychiatry.2017.3523.

Pérez-Vigil, A., Mittendorfer-Rutz, E., Helgesson, M., Brander, G., Isomura, K., Fernández de la Cruz, L., & Mataix-Cols, D. (2019). Labour market marginalisation in obsessive–compulsive disorder: A nationwide register-based sibling control study. *Psychological Medicine*, 49(1), 70–77. doi:10.1017/S0033291718001691.

Prato, A., Gulisano, M., Scerbo, M., & Barone, R. (2021). Diagnostic approach to pediatric autoimmune neuropsychiatric disorders associated with streptococcal infections (PANDAS): A narrative review of literature data. *Frontiers in Pediatrics*, 9, 746639. doi:10.3389/fped.2021.746639.

Salzman, L. (1980). *Understanding the obsessional personality.* New York: Jason Aronson.

Scahill, L., Riddle, M. A., McSwiggin-Hardin, M., Ort, S. I., King, R. A., Goodman, W. K., Cicchetti, D., & Leckman, J. F. (1997). Children's Yale-Brown Obsessive Compulsive Scale: Reliability and validity. *Journal of the American Academy of Child & Adolescent Psychiatry*, 36(6), 844–852. doi:10.1097/00004583-199706000-00023.

Sharp, C., & Wall, K. (2018). Personality development in adolescence. In O. P. John & R. W. Robins (Eds), *Handbook of personality: Theory and research* (4th ed., pp. 345–365). New York: Guilford Press.

Steele, D. W., Kanaan, G., Caputo, E. L., Freeman, J. B., Brannan, E. H., Balk, E. M., Trikalinos, T. A., & Adam, G. P. (2025). Treatment of obsessive-compulsive disorder in children and youth: A meta-analysis. *Pediatrics*, 155(3), doi:10.1542/peds.2024-068992.

Stiede, J. T., Spencer, S. D., & Onyeka, O. (2024). Obsessive–compulsive disorder in children and adolescents. *Annual Review of Clinical Psychology*, 20(1), 355–380, doi:10.1146/annurev-clinpsy-080822-043910.

Storch, E. A., McGuire, J. F., Wu, M. S., Hamblin, R., McIngvale, E., Cepeda, S. L., Schneider, S. C., Rufino, K. A., Rasmussen, S. A., Price, L. H., & Goodman, W. K. (2019). Development and psychometric evaluation of the Children's Yale-Brown Obsessive-Compulsive Scale Second Edition. *Journal of the American Academy of Child & Adolescent Psychiatry*, 58(1), 92–98. doi:10.1016/j.jaac.2018.05.029.

Subramanian, V., & Mayur, P. (2018). Trauma precursors of obsessive compulsive disorder: A case series. *International Journal of Depression & Anxiety*, doi:10.23937/ijda-2017/1710001.

van Steensel, F. J. A., Bögels, S. M., & Perrin, S. (2011). Anxiety disorders in children and adolescents with autistic spectrum disorders: A meta-analysis. *Clinical Child and Family Psychology Review*, 14(3), 302–317. doi:10.1007/s10567-011-0097-0.

Woods, E. E., & Gantt-Howrey, A. (2023). 'I'm So #OCD': A content analysis of how women portray OCD on TikTok. *The Professional Counselor*, 13(1), 27–43. doi:10.15241/eew.13.1.27.

World Health Organization (WHO). (2019). *International classification of diseases for mortality and morbidity statistics (11th revision)*. https://icd.who.int/.

Wu, M. S., Rudy, B. M., & Storch, E. A. (2014). Obsessions, compulsions, and repetitive behavior: Autism and/or OCD. In T. Davis III, S. White, & T. Ollendick (Eds), *Handbook of autism and anxiety* (pp. 153–168). New York: Springer. https://link.springer.com/chapter/10.1007/978-3-319-06796-4_8.

From Infancy to Intrusions

Early Mechanisms in Adolescent OCD

Obsessive-compulsive disorder (OCD) does not appear in adolescence without roots. What we encounter in the clinic, the intrusive thoughts, the worrying, the time-consuming compulsions, are often late echoes of mechanisms first used for survival in infancy. These are universal processes, deeply embodied and shaped long before they can be recognised, let alone understood.

In Chapter 2, I described what I called structural OCD, where early ways of coping seem to linger beneath the surface and later reappear with greater force. Parents will sometimes recall faint traces of these patterns in childhood, small rituals or worries that were dismissed as quirks and then seemed to fade. In adolescence, they return, intensified by new emotional pressures. Even in the more situational forms of OCD that emerge after a clear stressor, the mechanisms themselves are not new. They belong to infancy, to the earliest attempts to manage absence and uncertainty, and are simply reignited under fresh strain. In other words, whether an adolescent has a history of OCD-like behaviours or not, the mechanisms that underpin their OCD can be traced back to infancy.

These traces may be long forgotten in conscious memory, but they are not erased. As infants, long before personality or a sense of self has formed, we rely on primitive mental mechanisms to manage absence, frustration, and the flood of feelings we can neither name nor comprehend. Those early strategies, the illusion that a cry might summon milk or comfort, the division of the world into safe and unsafe, were adaptive then. In adolescence, under new pressures, they can return in distorted form, shaping obsessions and compulsions with a force that feels both archaic and immediate (Evans & Leckman, 2015; Brandchaft, 2001).

When adolescents sit in front of me in the consulting room, I often notice how these early mechanisms resurface under new strain. What once worked as protection begins to feel restrictive, and sometimes takes on a more ominous tone. A small fear that once steadied now torments; a familiar ritual that once soothed becomes worrying in its insistence.

I recall a 17-year-old who remembered always lining up her soft toys at the start of each day. As a child, she said this was 'for good luck', a memory her

DOI: 10.4324/9781003729716-3

mother also recalled. She grew out of it for a time, yet by 15 she found herself lining up anything she touched, no longer for good luck but to ward off bad luck. By 17 the ritual had spread so far that her movements were constrained and she had begun to withdraw into isolation. The fear of bad things happening had become so intense that avoidance and retreat felt safer than risk. Here was a concrete example of how an old way of coping, once harmless, had hardened into something distressing, shaping the fabric of her later adolescence.

In clinical terms, what we witness in such cases are not the sudden revelations of pathology but the return of older psychic residues. The omnipotent belief that actions can secure safety, once a creative adaptation in infancy, has re-emerged under the pressures of adolescence, now tinged with guilt and fear. The wish to control fortune, once playful, becomes a moral obligation. This shift marks the point where early magic turns into compulsion, where symbolic play loses its elasticity and hardens into ritual necessity.

These early psychic mechanisms are not pathological in themselves. They belong to ordinary infancy. Mechanisms such as omnipotence, splitting, repetition, and the illusion of control all serve a purpose in those first months of life. What makes them troubling later is not that they persist, but that they may develop in unusual ways or become so rigid that they weigh heavily on daily life. Careful infant observation has long suggested that even the youngest babies find ways of managing the anxieties of absence and frustration (Hall, Dwyer, & Magagna, 2019; Bozicevic et al., 2025). To those outside the psychoanalytic tradition, such descriptions of what infants do psychically to defend themselves can sound imaginative, yet the evidence is clear that the infant's inner life, however primitive, is active in defending itself. How these processes are understood and described will depend on the theoretical lens one adheres to. Yet one thing remains clear: the mind uses an array of mental mechanisms to survive, and it is these same mechanisms that later play a part in the development of OCD.

Modern developmental research may use different language, but the picture it paints is strikingly similar. Studies of emotion regulation show that when caregiver responsiveness is withdrawn, infants often cling to repetitive behaviours that echo splitting or the illusion of control, as if holding on to predictability in the face of rupture (Beebe & Lachmann, 1994; Hytroś-Kiwała & Dacka, 2025). These strategies are vital in the first months of life, but if they remain fixed or reappear in adolescence, they become the very patterns that tighten into distress.

What I keep returning to is that these residues are not signs of illness. Almost every adolescent brushes against magical thinking, the impulse to split the world in two, or the fleeting belief that thoughts alone can alter reality. It belongs to the turbulence of adolescence. I see it in ordinary sessions, and I remember it from my own adolescence too, that sudden certainty that an idea holds power, or the strange comfort of dividing things neatly into good and bad. Looking back, those moments were often ways of managing more complex feelings.

What sets these processes apart, and why they matter so much in this work, is what happens when they do not pass. For most young people, the intensity fades; it softens, becomes part of reflection, and is woven into their growing-up story. But for those who go on to develop OCD, the same habits stiffen. A boy who once ran around in a Spiderman cape feeling invincible later finds that sense of omnipotence turned into a trap. A girl who once loved daydreams finds herself terrified by intrusive thoughts of a 'virgin birth', caught replaying what she knows cannot be real yet she cannot dismiss.

I have sat with many young people at this point, hearing them say, often with frustration, 'I know it doesn't make sense, but I can't stop.' What was once an echo of early childhood becomes a cage in adolescence. That is the distinction I hold in mind: not whether these mechanisms exist – they do, in everyone – but whether they have turned rigid, repetitive, and unyielding. When they reach that point, OCD takes hold.

In this chapter, we go back in time, not historically but developmentally, to trace these early psychological mechanisms and explore how they echo in the adolescent mind. The previous chapter outlined how OCD is formally defined and assessed, along with the cultural and developmental factors that can support or distort its presentation. Here we turn beneath those definitions, following the residues of infancy that lie dormant until adolescence awakens them.

The idea that universal mechanisms from infancy might be linked to OCD came alive for me during a moment of clinical observation. I remember sitting as a trainee clinical psychologist with my supervisor while he assessed a young man recently diagnosed with OCD. Once the young person had settled, wearing a Marvel versus Capcom T-shirt that caught the eye, my supervisor asked if he liked Marvel comics. He nodded, and a short exchange followed about his favourite superheroes and what he admired in them. My supervisor then asked whether he had ever dressed up as one. The young man, embarrassed but smiling, admitted he had often pretended to be Spiderman as a child.

My supervisor observed that the same imaginative process was at work now as it had been then. In childhood, it had offered power, play, and a way of navigating a world ruled by adults. In adolescence, however, that same process had turned against him, fuelling anxiety and compulsions. Both the young person and I were struck by the resemblance, the same imaginative capacity, once protective, now imprisoning.

Before exploring each mechanism in detail, I find it useful to pause and ask: of all the processes that unfold in infancy, why these particular ones? The reason, I think, becomes clearer when we consider the struggles at the heart of OCD. The fear that thoughts can cause harm, the unbearable weight of responsibility, the urge to split the world into safe and unsafe, the compulsive pull of repetition, and the desperate attempt to control absence all echo patterns first seen in infancy. In adolescence, under the intensifying pressures of bodily change and moral awakening, these same patterns resurface, magnified and more troubling. They are not the only mechanisms shaping mental life, but in my experience they are the ones most consistently woven into obsessive and compulsive symptoms.

Empirical research within the cognitive tradition has also traced these developmental residues in later life. Constructs such as inflated responsibility, perfectionism, and intolerance of uncertainty, often identified as keeping processes in OCD (Pozza, Albert, & Dèttore, 2019; Reuther, Davis, & Rudy, 2013), can be understood as contemporary manifestations of the same early psychological mechanisms that once ensured psychic survival. The language differs, but both perspectives describe a similar process: adaptive efforts at control and certainty becoming rigid under stress.

I will begin by taking a developmental lens to these mechanisms. We start with those that emerge in the newborn's earliest days, the most primitive forms of psychic defence, and then move toward those that, while still rooted in infancy, develop a little later. This order is not rigid, but it helps trace how the earliest ways of coping give rise to more complex patterns that can reappear in adolescence.

Omnipotence of Thought

In the earliest months of life, we live in a world where thinking makes it so. Without conscious awareness, we believe we can control everything in a godlike manner. We wiggle in discomfort and warmth returns. We cry in hunger and food appears. The link feels immediate, as if wanting alone can make things happen. This is not a deliberate belief but an emotional reality, one that provides just enough security for growth to unfold.

Over time, small frustrations such as waiting to be fed or being left for a moment begin to show that the world is not fully under our control, and the mind slowly learns to bear that fact.

In adolescence, this early illusion often returns in a distorted way. A young person may feel that a violent image in their mind makes harm more likely, or that simply imagining a disaster is enough to bring it about. They know, rationally, that thoughts are not actions, yet the feeling insists otherwise. In infancy, this sense of omnipotence was never questioned; it was lived as fact, part of how the infant survived in a world too overwhelming to manage otherwise. In adolescence, under new pressures, the same process can turn against the young person, making the mind itself feel unsafe. Compulsions then emerge as desperate attempts to undo or neutralise these thoughts, as if safety could be restored by ritual alone. To show how this plays out in clinical practice, I will share two clinical examples.

I once worked with a 14-year-old boy who had stopped using sharp objects of any kind. He asked his parents to lock away knives, scissors, and even ordinary household tools. He explained that if a thought such as 'what if I stabbed my sister?' entered his mind, it might somehow make the act happen. He knew it was illogical, yet he remained convinced that simply having the thought made him dangerous. What he avoided was not the knife itself, but the destructive force he felt within his own mind. For him, the intrusive thought was lived as if it carried real power, echoing the unquestioned omnipotence of infancy now returned in distorted form.

I remember working through the sequence of actions with him, step by step, to show that for a thought to become an act a series of deliberate choices must take place. Together, we identified each stage that would be required, unpleasant as it was to picture such a violent act. In hindsight, it was a fruitful session; it planted the first seed of doubt about whether thoughts themselves truly possessed omnipotent power. Even so, I left with the uneasy sense that my words had not quite reached him, that the conviction of his omnipotent belief lay beyond the reach of purely behavioural or cognitive approaches.

I also recall a 16-year-old girl tormented by the conviction that she might somehow become pregnant despite never having been sexually active. Whenever a sexual image entered her mind, she would collapse into repetitive cycles of thought: 'I know it is impossible, but what if it happens?' She could explain rationally that this could not occur, yet the feeling insisted otherwise. At first glance, this fear of a 'virgin birth' seems a world apart from an infant crying in hunger and food appearing, yet the same mechanism is at work. In both cases, thought and reality collapse into one another. This is hard to grasp until you have sat with it in the room, but it is one of the key mechanisms in OCD. I see it again and again, whether with young people already diagnosed or with those whose obsessive and compulsive symptoms have not yet reached diagnostic threshold. The adolescent processes underneath – biological, sexual, and psychological – stir these early residues back into life, giving them a new and troubling force.

Wilfred Bion, writing in *Second Thoughts* (1967), particularly in his papers on schizophrenia, described how, in psychotic states, the boundaries between thought and action can disintegrate. Thinking becomes a substitute for doing, or doing replaces thinking altogether. Though the adolescents with OCD I see are far from psychotic, a similar confusion often colours their experience; thoughts feel performative, as if thinking were already doing.

In clinical practice, while this mechanism is related to most presentations of OCD, this specific mechanism most often reveals itself in harm, contamination, and sexual or moral obsessions: an adolescent convinced that thinking of a fire might make one start; another who avoids shaking hands in case a fleeting thought of 'infection' might somehow bring it about; or one who prays compulsively after a blasphemous image, fearing that mere imagination could damn them. Each variation carries the same underlying conviction that thoughts hold causal power.

From a psychoanalytic perspective, this mechanism is described as omnipotence of thought or, in more extreme states, megalomania. Many of my colleagues who work within a cognitive behavioural framework refer to it as thought action fusion. Both traditions are pointing to the same phenomenon, the collapse of the boundary between thought and reality. Whether we describe it as omnipotence or fusion, the adolescent experiences the mere presence of a thought as dangerous, binding, or predictive. Naming it differently does not change the fact that it sits at the very core of OCD, shaping both the fear itself and the compulsions that follow.

In my experience, however, thought action fusion, as described in the cognitive behavioural literature, often captures this only at the cognitive level. It lends itself to structured challenges and behavioural experiments, such as testing the assumption that thinking about an event will make it happen. This can be effective for some adolescents, and I use it myself at times. Yet, for others, even after completing these exercises, the terror remains. What I encounter in those cases feels more archaic, more entrenched, as though it were carried from a deeper layer of psychic life. This is where I draw a distinction between thought action fusion and omnipotence of thought. The former can be tested and corrected at the level of belief; the latter is harder to shift because it is not merely a mistaken idea but a residue of early experience that returns under the pressure of adolescence.

This is where, as I will discuss in later chapters, identifying the psychic position a young person is inhabiting in relation to their OCD symptoms becomes crucial. For instance, an adolescent in a more depressive position is often able to make use of behavioural challenges aimed at thought action fusion, engaging with the exercises in a way that feels meaningful. By contrast, those in more entrenched positions, such as the claustrum or the paranoid–schizoid position, may find such exercises irrelevant or complete them out of politeness, without any deeper connection. For these young people, the difficulty lies less in testing a belief than in loosening the archaic conviction that their thoughts themselves are dangerous.

It is important to recognise that while this mechanism originates in infancy, it re-emerges in adolescence with new force, shaped by the young person's internal relationship to their thoughts. That relationship in turn influences which interventions are likely to be effective. For some, behavioural experiments can loosen the grip of thought action fusion. For others, the archaic conviction of omnipotence requires slower, symbol-attuned work. Again and again, I am reminded that the task is not to choose one model over another but to integrate, to work with what is present in the room, and to tailor the approach accordingly.

If omnipotence of thought collapses the boundary between inner and outer, splitting tries to restore safety by drawing a harder line. Where one mechanism fuses thought with reality, the other divides experience into simple, protective categories of good and bad. Both aim to manage unmanageable feeling, but they do so in opposite ways. It is to this dividing move, and the costs it brings, that I now turn.

Splitting

Alongside omnipotent thought, another of the earliest ways the infant organises experience is through splitting (Klein, 1946). In the beginning, we are flooded by raw, nameless sensations, both from within and from the world around us (Bion, 1962). To remain connected, the infant needs a simple way to make sense of what is happening. If someone feeds, nurtures, and soothes, then in the earliest mind that same figure cannot also be the one who frustrates or disappears. Splitting protects against the terror of contradiction (Fairbairn, 1944; Freud, 1938/1941). At this stage, we cannot yet imagine that the same source of nourishment can both satisfy and disappoint. Instead, as Klein described, the world is divided into extremes of good and bad, loving and unloving, safe and unsafe.

Contradiction, for the infant, is unbearable not because it doesn't make sense but because it feels like the end of the world. In other words, it feels annihilatory. To rely on someone who provides both love and frustration exposes just how limited one's control really is, how utterly dependent one is on another's care. Splitting protects against that helplessness by dividing experience into good and bad, safe and unsafe. It is less a distortion than a survival strategy, a way of keeping hold of coherence when ambivalence would otherwise tear it apart.

If development unfolds in a 'good enough' environment (Winnicott, 1953), one where physical and emotional needs are met consistently though never perfectly, we begin to learn that our more negative feelings do not make us unlovable. The same parent who frustrates us can also be the one who loves us, and moments of anger or envy do not destroy that emotional bond. The capacity to live with ambivalence is a lifelong achievement, but a fragile one. It falters when we are stressed or afraid, and it often falters again in adolescence.

So many experiences at this stage are new, and outside the young person's control: social popularity, academic success, the bodily transformations of puberty. The skill of carrying ambivalence is still developing. This is why splitting so often resurfaces in these years as a way to manage the overwhelming uncertainty that comes with new experiences and shifting identities. I will illustrate this by reflecting on several clinical examples.

I saw this vividly in a 16-year-old who told me, with absolute conviction, that separating things into contaminated and not contaminated was the only way he could feel safe. Anything he touched after an angry thought about his parents became dirty: his football kit, his books, even his schoolbag. For a long time, we circled around illness and hygiene, but in time it became clear that what looked like cleanliness was really a desperate attempt to ward off harm, especially the fear of being attacked or rejected by others.

I have seen the same process in different guises. One girl felt compelled to confess every angry thought she had toward her younger brother, fearing that not doing so meant she was secretly dangerous to him. Another could not wear certain clothes after thinking of a sexual image, as if the thought had stained them beyond repair. In both cases, the compulsion was less about germs or morality in any straightforward sense, and more about an inability to hold love and hate, purity and corruption, safety and danger together. Splitting made the world feel more manageable, even if at great personal cost.

From a psychoanalytic perspective, these compulsions can be understood as rigid defences against the terror of ambivalence. In other words, the idea of tolerating uncertainty and acknowledging more complex or mixed feelings feels too unsafe. Contemporary cognitive behavioural models describe something similar in terms of intolerance of uncertainty and overestimation of threat. Whether we call it splitting or intolerance of uncertainty, the problem is the same. The adolescent cannot bear the messiness of mixed states, so rituals arise to keep the world divided into clear categories of safe and unsafe, good and bad.

In the consulting room, the task is not to strip rituals away too quickly but to help the adolescent experiment with holding contradictory experiences without rushing to repair them. This may mean tolerating an object that feels contaminated by a bad thought, or noticing that a moment of anger does not erase love. At times, my role is to model ambivalence directly in the room, naming both sides of the conflict and allowing them to sit together. For example, I have found it useful to say something like, 'I can see that part of you is furious with her, and another part loves her deeply. Both can be true.'

It can be especially difficult to tolerate uncertainty during adolescence, when so much else already feels unstable. Physical change, sexual development, shifting peer relationships, and academic pressure all heighten the sense of unpredictability. Against this backdrop, OCD offers the illusion of certainty by splitting the world into safe and unsafe, pure and contaminated. The work of therapy is to help the young person discover, slowly, that uncertainty can be survived, even in the midst of turbulence.

From a cognitive behavioural therapy (CBT) perspective, exposure and response prevention (ERP) is often used to target this process. By helping young people stay with feelings of contamination or uncertainty without acting on rituals, ERP can gradually build tolerance for ambivalence. I cover this in more detail in Chapter 6, where I look at the strengths and limits of ERP in practice. Here, it is enough to note that, as with other interventions, its impact depends on the psychic position the adolescent occupies. For some adolescents, particularly those able to reflect and engage from a more depressive position (Chapter 11), ERP can be effective and even transformative. For others in more entrenched positions, such as the claustrum (Chapter 8) or the paranoid–schizoid position (Chapter 10), ERP may be attempted but has little emotional impact. They may complete the tasks yet remain terrified underneath.

To work with splitting in adolescence is to sit close to the longing for certainty, while also holding open the possibility that love and hate, safety and danger, can be carried together.

We often encourage adolescents to 'take responsibility', as if it were a rite of passage. Yet the roots of responsibility run deeper, reaching back into infancy. As babies, we live with the fantasy that our thoughts shape the world. We begin to feel that the emotions we cannot control might harm those we depend on. At this stage, there is no conscious capacity to think in this way. It is a felt experience, one that precedes logical thought, carried in the body and emotions rather than in words or ideas. A caregiver who withdraws under the strain of a baby's cries, or who becomes anxious in the face of distress, may leave behind a trace of fear. This can translate into a message for the baby: my feelings are too much; they can drive you away.

These early impressions, while not stored in conscious memory, do not simply vanish. Adolescence brings a new wave of responsibility. There is a natural push toward independence, greater ownership, and a reshaping of relationships within the family. Physiological change is part of this. A boy who grows taller, develops facial hair and muscle, may suddenly be treated as more capable. He is expected to do more on his own and to protect others. His physique now carries the potential to do real damage to those he loves, unlike the 2-year-old version of himself whose aggressive impulses could be safely contained by an adult. For girls, the changes of puberty can shift family dynamics in another way. As breasts and other secondary sexual characteristics emerge, a father may unconsciously step back from direct care, treating her less as a child and more as a young woman. The responsibility placed on her increases, often before she feels ready.

In the clinic, I often see how these developmental shifts intensify the burden of responsibility and find expression in obsessive-compulsive symptoms. A 16-year-old boy, convinced it would be his fault if anything happened overnight, checked every door and socket in the house before bed. A girl of the same age checked the stove and windows, certain her parents would die in their sleep if she did not. What looked from the outside like ordinary caution was in fact the crushing sense that they alone were responsible for keeping everyone safe.

This mechanism may resemble omnipotence of thought, but there is a key distinction. Omnipotence fears that thoughts themselves are dangerous; responsibility fears that failing to act will leave others unprotected. Both place the adolescent in an impossible position.

From a cognitive behavioural perspective, interventions such as behavioural experiments and responsibility reattribution can help loosen this bias.

One practical method, sometimes called the responsibility pie chart, invites the adolescent to visualise how many other factors contribute to feared outcomes beyond their control. Similar re-apportioning techniques are described in CBT manuals for OCD (Sperry & Sperry, 2017; Salkovskis, 1999; Wilhelm & Steketee, 2006). The exercise is not a cure in itself, but when used thoughtfully it can be a gentle way of loosening rigid responsibility beliefs. Its usefulness, however, depends greatly on the psychic position the young person occupies. For those in a more depressive position, these tasks can be meaningful and bring real relief. For those in more entrenched positions, such as the claustrum or the paranoid–schizoid, the exercises may be completed politely but without deeper impact. Here, the felt burden of responsibility is less a mistaken belief than a survival strategy rooted in early experience, and work must proceed at that level if it is to make a difference.

Other therapeutic approaches have also shown value in addressing inflated responsibility. Acceptance and commitment therapy (ACT) supports adolescents in noticing and stepping back from their thoughts rather than engaging in a struggle to control them. This shift in stance can reduce the emotional weight of intrusive thoughts and compulsions, and has shown promising results in youth populations (Armstrong, Morrison, & Twohig, 2013). Inference-based therapy (IBT), although not yet supported by published studies specifically focused on adolescents at the time of writing, speaks directly to responsibility beliefs. It guides individuals to examine the leap from doubt to certainty that often fuels compulsive behaviours (Julien, O'Connor, & Aardema, 2016).

These approaches, supported by emerging empirical findings, demonstrate that there is more than one route to change. My view is that all of these interventions can be, and for some young people truly are, effective. Yet before any of them can reach their full impact, we must remain mindful of the psychic position the adolescent holds in relation to their OCD. Without that, even the best-designed technique will miss its mark.

Repetition, Symmetry, and Mastery

A 14-year-old boy once told me that if he did not tap each side of his body an equal number of times, he felt as though he might explode. He laughed nervously as he described it, admitting he knew nothing bad would actually happen, but the feeling of imbalance was unbearable. He said it was all-consuming, as if he could not be fully human unless he completed the ritual. Another adolescent spent hours arranging objects on her desk until they looked 'just right'. If anyone moved them, she would rush to fix them, insisting it was not about order or neatness but about an inside feeling that would not settle otherwise. She often began our sessions by complaining about how unreasonable her mother was for attempting to clean or even shift things in her room.

In adolescence this pull toward balance often returns with force. For some young people it is not about fearing catastrophe but about chasing a sense of being 'just right'. They describe it as an inner dissonance, as if life itself cannot move forward until symmetry is restored. I have sat with adolescents who could not leave the house until their shoes were perfectly aligned, or who tapped both shoulders equally because leaving one side out felt unbearable. For parents, this can be especially difficult to understand. Unlike contamination fears, there is often no clear feared outcome. The fear is not of germs or harm but of being unable to settle until the uneasy feeling has passed.

A 15-year-old boy once told me how, every night before bed, he had to switch his lamp on and off exactly 21 times. He laughed awkwardly as he explained it, insisting he knew it was pointless, that nothing bad would happen if he stopped. Yet the longer we talked, the more obvious it became how trapped he felt. If he lost count or made a mistake, he had to begin again, sometimes for half an hour or more. It was the only way he could feel settled enough to sleep. Sitting with him, I felt the weight of how joyless the ritual had become. It carried none of the playfulness or flexibility that repetition usually holds in childhood. It was work, and he knew it, but he could not stop.

Another adolescent, a 13-year-old girl, told me she had to go up and down the stairs an even number of times before bed. Some nights it was 12, others 36, and occasionally just 4. When I asked why the number changed, she shrugged. She did not know, only that it had to feel right. What struck me was how matter of fact she was, almost as if she were reporting a rule rather than describing a symptom. If I had pressed her too quickly for meaning, she would have felt unsafe and probably left therapy altogether. So we stayed with it as it was. For her, the act of repeating was not about numbers at all but about safety, and stopping felt impossible.

As babies, we are also naturally drawn to repetition. We drop toys from the high chair again and again, babble strings of syllables, or play peekaboo with delight. These repetitions are not problematic behaviours but the beginnings of mastery. They are how helplessness is transformed into a sense of influence. To understand how this happens, it helps to return to the origins of repetition itself. Before it becomes a symptom, repetition is a way of making sense of absence and return, of discovering that what disappears might come back. It is the first form of hope, enacted through rhythm.

Freud described the fort-da game, where a child repeatedly threw and retrieved a spool to master the anxiety of absence. Perhaps a spool is not as exciting nowadays, but the principle is the same. My own daughter at 18 months would stack magnetic blocks into a tower, knock it down, and then look at me for a smile and applause before rebuilding it. Repetition continues as we grow. Adolescents rehearse for exams, repeat strategies at football and rugby training, or study notes again and again. These forms of repetition build competence and confidence. They are flexible, purposeful, and adaptive.

In OCD, however, repetition loses this flexibility. It becomes fixated and devoid of pleasure, stripped of its link to mastery and success. The adolescent repeats not to learn or to play but to ward off catastrophe. The door must be locked, not once but ten times. Hands must be washed, not until clean but until they feel right. What began as an adaptive developmental process becomes arrested, trapping the adolescent in cycles that shrink their world rather than expand it.

Parents sometimes dismiss compulsions as just habits, but in OCD the quality of repetition is different. It is not about practice or pleasure but about neutralising an internal sense of dread. For many adolescents, the compulsion continues not because they believe something bad will happen, but because it does not yet feel right to stop. This feeling of incompleteness or wrongness, often referred to in the literature as Not Just Right Experience, is a well-established feature in OCD research. I can reflect on many experiences with adolescents who have described to me this internal push to keep doing something until it feels just right. This is thought of as a core feature of their difficulties, and research suggests it is closely linked to symptom severity, particularly in young people (Cervin & Borrelli, 2025). They are not simply quirks or preferences, but deeply felt emotional states that compel action until relief is achieved.

The therapeutic task is to help the adolescent rediscover flexibility, to experiment with stopping, delaying, or altering rituals, and to learn that the feared consequences do not occur, or that the feeling of wrongness can be tolerated. In CBT, this may take the form of exposure with response prevention. In more relational work, it may involve exploring the dread beneath the repetition and gradually strengthening the adolescent's capacity to bear it without ritual.

From a cognitive behavioural perspective, exposure work often targets this very pattern by asking the adolescent to resist or delay their repetitive ritual. For some, particularly those able to reflect from a more depressive position, such exercises can loosen the grip of repetition and bring real relief. For others in more entrenched positions, such as the claustrum, psychic retreat, or the paranoid–schizoid, the tasks may be carried out but without deeper effect. They may comply outwardly yet remain terrified underneath. In these cases, repetition is not simply a habit to be broken but a survival strategy that has become rigid. Recognising the psychic position helps us to know when exposure can be effective and when it must be carefully integrated into a broader therapeutic stance.

To sit with an adolescent caught in repetition is to feel both the longing for safety and the cost of rigidity. The task of therapy is not only to break the cycle but to help them rediscover the freedom that repetition once gave – the play, the mastery, the delight – and to carry some of that forward into adolescence.

Contamination and Purity

Not all the processes that shape OCD in adolescence can be traced back to a single mechanism rooted in infancy. Some are better understood as developmental themes: patterns that emerge early and shift over time. I believe contamination and purity fall into this category. These experiences do not arise from one psychic structure but from a constellation of early moments linking the body, emotion, and morality. Though perhaps less subtle than intrapsychic mechanisms like omnipotence or splitting, the theme of contamination is no less powerful. As you may have gathered from the clinical material I have shared, it is one of the most common and deeply distressing dimensions of OCD. Its roots run deep.

This symbolic layering of contamination came into sharper focus during my work with a 12-year-old boy who told me he needed to shower three times every night. The first shower, he said, was to get rid of 'normal dirt'. The second was for 'the germs that people carry'. The third, he explained, was to wash away 'the bad feelings from the day'. I asked how he knew when those feelings had gone, and he paused before saying, 'I just don't feel disgusting anymore.' His parents assumed he was simply particular about hygiene, maybe even proud of his appearance. But, over time, it became clear that the ritual had far less to do with cleanliness and much more to do with purging an internal sense of pollution.

As infants, our earliest experiences are entangled with feeding, weaning, and soiling. Bodily care brings comfort and relief, but also discomfort and sometimes disgust. Toilet training introduces a charged moment when control over the body starts to become associated with pride, shame, and the emerging sense of being good or bad. Disgust sensitivity, already present early on, is shaped further by parental responses and broader culture (Tybur et al., 2018). By adolescence, these residues return, often with new symbolic force. Dirt and germs are no longer just physical concerns; they come to represent inner corruption, weakness, or danger. In more overt social terms, a child seen as 'dirty' at school may be labelled a loner, unpleasant, or unpopular. The meaning of dirt extends well beyond the literal and into the social sphere, where it can isolate a young person. And it often extends even further into the realm of internal experience, as the next example illustrates.

At this point, one can appreciate that such an interpretation might feel adrift to those trained primarily in behavioural or cognitive approaches. From those perspectives, contamination fears may appear as learned associations or misinterpretations of bodily sensations. That layer certainly exists, and it is a useful one to hold in mind. Yet what I am proposing here is that these behaviours stand still for something deeper. Beneath the surface conditioning, they are attempts to manage unbearable feelings of moral or emotional pollution, states that words have not yet reached. We can see echoes of this far beyond the clinic. Across literature, myth, and even the small dramas of modern life, people scrub at guilt, rewash clothes, or bathe after betrayal, as if cleansing the body might absolve the mind. Such images remind us that the wish to wash away psychic stain is not confined to pathology; it is part of the wider human effort to purify what feels spoiled.

I once worked with a 16-year-old girl who scrubbed her body raw after certain social interactions. It took months for either of us to realise that these were the moments in which she had felt humiliated or criticised. What those situations stirred in her was anger: intense, unacknowledged, and impossible to express. She had grown up believing that anger was immature and unacceptable. For her, it was especially unacceptable in girls. She carried an unquestioned belief that female anger was ugly, even shameful. So, rather than acknowledge it, she washed it away. What looked, on the surface, like obsessive hygiene turned out to be a desperate effort to rid herself of feelings she could not tolerate.

Compulsive cleaning is rarely about hygiene alone. More often, it is an attempt to manage overwhelming feelings such as disgust, shame, or a sense of moral contamination that may feel imagined but is no less real in its emotional impact. Parents sometimes misread the behaviour as maturity or assume it reflects strong personal preferences. When praised or left unchecked, the rituals often gain quiet momentum. The distress involved can be so intense that it may take adolescents several sessions, sometimes much longer, before they are able to name what is really going on. A small number of those who have presented with compulsive washing, particularly around personal hygiene, have eventually shared that wet dreams, or for girls the confusing physical changes tied to arousal or occasional nocturnal orgasm, are deeply distressing. Even when they know such responses are biologically normal, the shame can be overwhelming. Often there is a disconnection, almost a denial, of the adolescent body itself. At times, it feels eerily similar to a 2-year-old struggling with the emotional implications of toilet training.

In families, contamination rituals rarely exist in isolation. Parents often find themselves drawn in to the same anxious system. I have worked with families who began buying endless quantities of soap, shower gel, and disinfectant, at first to support a growing child's developing body, but soon to manage a deeper, unnamed dread. What begins as care quietly reinforces the ritual. In other homes, parents withdraw in frustration, unable to watch their child scrub themselves raw. Both reactions, anxious participation or weary retreat, make sense, yet each risks confirming the adolescent's sense of danger or badness. The contamination spreads beyond the sink or shower; it seeps into the family atmosphere. Part of the therapeutic work, often early on, is helping parents tolerate their own helplessness without turning it into action.

In therapy, the task is not to debate hygiene or insist on logical thinking. It is to create enough space for the adolescent to begin naming the feelings beneath the surface. From a CBT standpoint, this connects directly with exposure and response prevention, helping the young person stay with feelings like shame or disgust without falling into ritual. From a relational perspective, the work is about creating enough safety for those buried feelings to emerge in the first place. In both approaches, the goal is not to eliminate the impulse to cleanse but to loosen its grip and, in doing so, to support a more integrated and compassionate relationship with the self.

Magical Thinking and the Illusion of Control

A 17-year-old girl told me that if she did not silently repeat a certain phrase every night before bed, her family would die in their sleep. She admitted she knew it made no sense but said, 'I just can't take the risk.' Another young person explained that whenever he thought something bad might happen, he had to cross his fingers until the thought passed. He laughed at how childish it sounded, then added quietly, 'It still feels real.'

As children, magical thinking is part of ordinary development. We put on a cape and believe we have become a superhero. We avoid stepping on cracks in the pavement to keep bad luck away. These small rituals help us feel powerful in a world where so much is out of our control. As I described earlier when observing my supervisor, the same imaginative process that once allowed a boy to feel powerful as Spiderman returned in adolescence as something frightening and imprisoning. What was once playful became persecutory. For most children, magical thinking softens as reasoning develops and the world becomes more predictable, but in some adolescents it returns with force, now bound to fear rather than play.

What makes magical thinking so powerful is not its logic but its feeling. The act of repeating, touching, or crossing fingers translates an invisible dread into something that can be managed. It gives anxiety a form. This is often a clinician's Achilles heel. The young person may fully acknowledge the irrationality and absence of belief in their magical thinking, yet the feeling remains too real. In moments like this it is easy to get pulled into abstract arguments or philosophies of logic, when what is often most helpful, again depending on the psychic position the young person occupies in relation to their OCD, is to stay with that frightening discrepancy between what one believes and what one feels.

It also seems to mark a transitional space between early omnipotence and the later emergence of moral responsibility. The adolescent is no longer a child who believes their thoughts create reality, yet not fully an adult who can bear that reality unfolds beyond their control. Magical thinking fills that gap, allowing agency to be felt where it might otherwise be lost. It restores a sense of influence at precisely the point where helplessness feels most intolerable.

There is a close link here with what I described earlier about omnipotence of thought and inflated responsibility. Magical thinking sits nearest to omnipotence, where thoughts are experienced as powerful in themselves, yet it often carries the flavour of responsibility when the ritual is framed as protecting others. The adolescent may know that repeating a phrase cannot literally keep their family safe, yet the felt conviction is that not doing it would be a kind of neglect. In this way, omnipotence, responsibility, and magical thinking overlap, but they remain distinct enough to be clinically useful.

Clinically, these presentations can look strange from the outside, but in the room they make sense. They are attempts to manage overwhelming anxiety with the only tools available. For some adolescents, behavioural experiments that test whether the feared outcome occurs can help loosen the grip of magical thinking. For others, especially those in more entrenched psychic positions, these rituals are less about mistaken beliefs and more about surviving unbearable states of mind. In those cases, therapy must first attend to the fear underneath before rituals can safely be relinquished.

Even adults are not immune to magical thinking. We touch wood before a journey or avoid saying something out loud for fear of tempting fate. These small superstitions are diluted remnants of the same process. In adolescence, they re-emerge in sharper form, no longer hidden beneath social convention but lived in the open, where they can cause real suffering.

To sit with magical thinking is to see the double edge of imagination. The same faculty that once gave a child freedom and play can, in adolescence, bind them to rituals that feel life or death. The task of therapy is not to strip away imagination but to help the adolescent carry it differently, so that its power can return to creativity rather than fear.

Conclusion

What I have tried to show in this chapter is that the OCD symptoms we meet in adolescence are not random intrusions or compulsions that suddenly appear. They are elaborations of early psychic and developmental mechanisms seen in all infants. Omnipotent thought, inflated responsibility, splitting, repetition, and magical control once safeguarded survival. They helped the infant manage absence, uncertainty, and raw feeling. By adolescence, under the strain of physical change, new sexuality, shifting relationships, and the demands of growing thought, these same processes return in more elaborate and often troubling ways.

Recognising these continuities matters. It shows that compulsions are not meaningless habits but the latest forms of strategies that once worked. It reminds us to pitch our interventions to the psychic position the young person holds, and to draw on different therapeutic traditions rather than set them against one another. Above all, it lets us meet the adolescent not as a collection of symptoms but as someone trying to survive development with the tools they have to hand.

I find this way of thinking offers both compassion and precision. It allows us to see the symbolic purpose within even the most bewildering rituals, to look at what the symptom is protecting rather than simply what it is preventing. It is a stance that keeps curiosity alive when progress stalls, and that guards us, as clinicians, against the pull to tidy away complexity too soon.

If infancy provides the roots, adolescence provides the storm. The next chapter turns directly to that turbulence, with its surge of sexual and aggressive impulses, the awakening of morality, and the collision of these forces with intrusive thought. If this chapter has been about the ground beneath the symptom, the next is about the weather above it, how those same roots are shaken when adolescence arrives in full force.

Seen in this way, OCD in adolescence is not a fixed category or an isolated disorder but a moving structure shaped by time, relationship, and growth. This way of looking invites an integrative stance, one that holds both the evidence base of cognitive treatments and the symbolic depth of analytic thought. My hope is that, in holding these together, our understanding of OCD becomes a little more human, a little closer to the young people who live it.

References

Armstrong, A. B., Morrison, K. L., & Twohig, M. P. (2013). A preliminary investigation of acceptance and commitment therapy for adolescent obsessive-compulsive disorder. *Journal of Cognitive Psychotherapy*, 27(2), 175–190. doi:10.1891/0889-8391.27.2.175.

Beebe, B., & Lachmann, F. M. (1994). Representation and internalization in infancy: Three principles of salience. *Psychoanalytic Psychology*, 11(2), 127–165. doi:10.103 7/h0079530.

Bion, W. R. (1962). A theory of thinking. *International Journal of Psycho-Analysis*, 43, 1–23.

Bion, W. R. (1967). *Second thoughts: Selected papers on psychoanalysis* (1st ed.). London and New York: Routledge. doi:10.4324/9780429479809.

Bozicevic, L., De Pascalis, L., Cooper, P., & Murray, L. (2025). The role of maternal sensitivity, infant temperament, and emotional context in the development of emotion regulation. *Scientific Reports*, 15(1), article 17271. doi:10.1038/s41598-025-01714-8.

Brandchaft, B. (2001). Obsessional disorders: A developmental systems perspective. *Psychoanalytic Inquiry*, 21(3), 321–340. doi:10.1080/07351692109348935.

Cervin, M., & Borrelli, D. F. (2025). Incompleteness and not just right experiences in children and adolescents with obsessive-compulsive disorder. In E. A. Storch & J. S. Abramowitz (Eds), *A clinician's guide to childhood obsessive-compulsive and related disorders* (pp. 17–32). London and New York: Routledge. doi:10.4324/9781003517429-4.

Evans, D. W., & Leckman, J. (2015). Origins of obsessive–compulsive disorder: Developmental and evolutionary perspectives. In J. Abramowitz, D. McKay, & E. Storch (Eds), *The Wiley handbook of obsessive compulsive disorders* (Vol. 1, pp. 133–152). Chichester: Wiley. doi:10.1002/9780470939406.ch10.

Fairbairn, W. R. D. (1944). Endopsychic structure considered in terms of object-relationships. *International Journal of Psycho-Analysis*, 25, 70–93.

Freud, S. (1938/1941). Splitting of the ego in the process of defence. In J. Strachey (Ed. & Trans.), *The standard edition of the complete psychological works of Sigmund Freud* (Vol. 23, pp. 271–278). London: Hogarth Press.

Hall, D., Dwyer, J., & Magagna, J. (2019). Separating from mother and saying goodbye to the infant observer. *Infant Observation: International Journal of Infant Observation and Its Applications*, 22(2–3),105–119. doi:10.1080/13698036.2019.1691625.

Hytroś-Kiwała, A., & Dacka, M. (2025). *Infant mental health: A developmental and psychoanalytic perspective. Psychoterapia*, 202(2), 67–81. https://www.psychoterap iaptp.pl/pdf-201182-126894?filename=126894.pdf.

Julien, D., O'Connor, K., & Aardema, F. (2016). The inference-based approach to obsessive-compulsive disorder: A comprehensive review of its etiological model, treatment efficacy, and model of change. *Journal of Affective Disorders*, 202, 187–196. doi:10.1016/j.jad.2016.05.060.

Klein, M. (1946). Notes on some schizoid mechanisms. *International Journal of Psycho-Analysis*, 27(3–4), 99–110.

Pozza, A., Albert, U., & Dèttore, D. (2019). Perfectionism and intolerance of uncertainty are predictors of OCD symptoms in children and early adolescents: A prospective, cohort, one-year, follow-up study. *Child Neuropsychiatry*, 16(1), 53–62. doi:10.1007/s00787-018-01248-4.

Reuther, E. T., Davis, T. E., & Rudy, B. M. (2013). Intolerance of uncertainty as a mediator of the relationship between perfectionism and obsessive–compulsive symptom severity. *Depression and Anxiety*, 30 (8), 773–777. doi:10.1002/da.22100.

Salkovskis, P. M. (1999). Understanding and treating obsessive–compulsive disorder. *Behaviour Research and Therapy*, 37(S1), S29–S52. doi:10.1016/S0005-7967(99)00049–00042.

Sperry, J., & Sperry, L. (2017). *Cognitive behavior therapy in counseling practice.* London and New York: Routledge. doi:10.4324/9781315626284.

Tybur, J. M., Çınar, Ç., Karinen, A. K., & Perone, P. (2018). Why do people vary in disgust? *Philosophical Transactions of the Royal Society B: Biological Sciences*, 373 (1751), 20170204. doi:10.1098/rstb.2017.0204.

Wilhelm, S., & Steketee, G. (2006). *Cognitive therapy for obsessive–compulsive disorder: A guide for professionals.* Oakland, CA: New Harbinger.

Winnicott, D. W. (1953). Transitional objects and transitional phenomena. *International Journal of Psycho-Analysis*, 34, 89–97.

Chapter 4

From Childhood Shadows to Adolescent Storms

Up to this point, I have often alluded to the intensity and radical transformation of adolescence itself. What I want to do now is look more closely, almost surgically, at what it is about this developmental stage that makes the mind so vulnerable to obsessional processes. If the last chapter showed how early psychic structures reappear in adolescence and take on the form of obsessive-compulsive disorder (OCD), this one turns to what it is within adolescence – its storms, its conflicts, its new capacities – that awakens them. To begin, we must think of adolescence not as a fixed period but as a process. While it is beyond the scope of this chapter to provide an exhaustive review of adolescent development, I will offer a selective survey of what I feel are the most crucial aspects that may provide a pathway to understanding why this is such a vulnerable time for obsessive-compulsive symptoms to develop.

Adolescence is not simply a continuation of childhood; it is a developmental upheaval driven by interacting biological, sociocultural, and psychological factors. To borrow and expand upon Meltzer and Harris (1986), adolescence can be thought of as a metaphorical process of renovation, a redesign of an existing structure in the mind, one created in infancy and solidified during latency. During the latent years, roughly between 6 and 11, rituals and magical thinking often soften, held by the relative stability of school life and by good enough experiences with people outside the family. This is usually a period when the more primitive and powerful emotions lie dormant. The mind's energy is invested elsewhere, in navigating friendships, acquiring knowledge, and developing practical and cognitive skills.

With puberty, as Winnicott (1963) observed, the young person enters the doldrums, a turbulent state in which dependence and independence are constantly battled over. Anna Freud (1958) noted how difficult it can be to distinguish ordinary upheaval from emerging mental disturbance at this stage. Early residues such as splitting, magical thinking, and omnipotence return with new urgency, reshaped by sexuality, bodily change, and moral awakening. What once protected the child can now imprison the adolescent and obstruct development. Freud (1905/1953) wrote that during this period, intense feelings linked to sexuality and morality can overwhelm the young

DOI: 10.4324/9781003729716-4

person's capacity to contain or make sense of them. In other words, the realisation of a sexualised body can stir confusion and anxiety.

A developing sense of right and wrong also becomes more complex and less certain than in earlier years, and this uncertainty itself can cause distress. My clinical experience supports these early psychoanalytic observations. Adolescents today still wrestle with the same dilemmas, and the turbulence described by Freud, Winnicott, and others continues to echo in the consulting room.

What has changed, however, is the world in which these struggles unfold. The social, cultural, and political climate has evolved enormously, from the ethics and etiquette of online communication to the wide spectrum of sexual and gender identities that adolescents must now navigate, accept, or reject. Expectations of what is considered normal or progressive have shifted in ways that are almost unrecognisable compared with my own adolescence in the 2000s, let alone Freud's and Winnicott's time.

Bion (1970) went further still, describing that, when thoughts cannot be processed, they can build up inside the mind and be experienced almost as an internal swelling or pressure. There are many ways to read Bion's statement, but, for me, he is describing what happens when the young person is newly inducted into thinking about things in a deeper and more personal way. It is the sudden awareness of having to think about oneself and to see the less desirable parts, to face them rather than hide behind action or denial. It also means having to tolerate frustration, to sit with not knowing, and to bear the uncertainty of who one is becoming and how others may change in response.

From a more contemporary perspective, neuroscience lends some context. The prefrontal cortex, responsible for reflective thought and impulse control, continues to mature well into the mid-twenties (Johnson, Blum, & Giedd, 2009 ; Mercurio et al., 2020). This biology helps explain why thoughts at this stage can feel immediate, overwhelming, and not easily contained by reason alone. The developmental mind is still learning how to think about itself without being swept away by the process.

In clinical practice, these perspectives resonate. Work with adolescents rarely follows a predictable path, despite the neat optics and pathways that services often present to the outside world. One session may bring genuine connection; the next may dissolve into silence, dismissal, or contempt. Progress can be undone in moments, which can feel both disappointing and frustrating for both the young person and the clinician. The same topic that feels light or even playful one week can return the next weighed down with shame, grief, or rage. This oscillation between openness and withdrawal, vitality and despair, belongs to the very nature of adolescence itself. It is a rhythm observed by psychotherapists across decades and cultures, regardless of theoretical orientation or clinical setting. Writers from Anderson and Dartington (1998) to Midgley et al. (2021), Oliveira, Ribeiro, and Gonçalves (2020), and most recently Sikand and Bhola (2024), have all described the same phenomenon in the consulting room: the adolescent mind as a landscape of approach and retreat, a continual testing of emotional contact and distance.

In my experience supervising clinicians from a range of backgrounds, many are candid enough to admit that they often shy away from working with adolescents because of the sheer emotional intensity they bring. Yet that same intensity is what makes the work so alive. The consulting room can feel volatile, charged with change, but it is within that volatility that obsessional symptoms often take shape. When the young person's inner world is in flux, the mind turns instinctively to whatever promises stability, even if that stability takes the form of debilitating obsessive or compulsive patterns. The same turbulence that makes adolescence so difficult also makes it creative: it is where both pathology and growth are fought over, often in the same breath.

When intrusive thoughts arise in this context, they rarely travel alone. They almost always arrive paired with compulsions, which show us how the adolescent is trying to survive the thought. I often think about adolescents who are coming into emotional contact with their sexuality or emerging sexual identity. They may defend against these new and confusing experiences through the manifestation of obsessive-compulsive symptoms. A 16-year-old girl once told me she could not leave the shower until her mind was free of sexual images. Each time a thought returned, she scrubbed harder, convinced that stepping out 'unclean' meant she was bad or corrupt. Her ritual was not about hygiene in any ordinary sense but about purging impulses she could not yet bear to claim as her own.

This example runs parallel with the moral dimension of sexuality that often emerges in adolescence, where thoughts about being a paedophile, a sex offender, or having inappropriate relationships take centre stage. The outward forms differ, but the underlying function is often the same. Over time, I have come to feel that such obsessions are attempts to defend against the anxiety created when pleasure and morality collide. The pleasurable instinct intersects with a developing moral consciousness, giving rise to thoughts of the worst possible sexual act one can imagine. The content may change, from fears of impregnating a family member to fantasies of being a predator, but the underlying struggle remains constant: a desperate effort to separate desire from danger, to make the intolerable bearable through ritual.

What is apparent, and likely very noticeable now, is that compulsions in adolescents carry a weight and burden different from the gestures of childhood. Magical control, repetition, and reassurance return under the pressures of puberty, sexuality, and moral development, but now with urgency and secrecy. What once looked like harmless play becomes burdened with guilt and shame. For the adolescent, these mechanisms are no longer protective games of mastery but prisons of survival.

When I think back over the adolescents I have worked with, what strikes me is the shifting trajectory of their intrusive thoughts. In structural OCD (see Chapter 2) – that is, OCD that emerges in childhood that may go completely unrecognised – the content often evolves across childhood, moving from fears of harm to the self, to worries about a parent's death, to anxieties about illness or contamination. With puberty, however, the themes often mutate. Intrusions take on a more violent or sexual quality, or circle around questions of sexual orientation. As I outlined earlier, not all repetitive behaviours at this stage are compulsions, but here I focus specifically on how intrusive thoughts and compulsions change in meaning during adolescence.

By adolescence, the inner landscape has altered. The mind can now imagine future scenarios, anticipate consequences, and grapple with questions of identity, sexuality, and morality. Childhood rituals that once linked action to safety are reinterpreted in this new light. These transformations are not random. They reveal how early mechanisms are reworked by puberty and moral awakening, gaining a force that is both recognisably adolescent and clinically troubling.

These shifts are not abstract. They arrive in the room with startling force. She is 16, silent, staring at the floor. Her mother has stepped out at her request. When she finally speaks, her voice is low, almost swallowed by shame: 'Sometimes I think I've done something … sexual … to my little brother. I haven't. I know I haven't. But it won't go away.' In that moment, the room holds both her terror and the storm of adolescence itself, where sexuality, morality, and the fear of losing control collide in thought.

OCD in adolescence sits at the centre of this turbulence. For some, it is the continuation of earlier patterns, the 'childhood shadows' of rituals and fears now taking on more symbolic weight. For others, it erupts suddenly, as if developmental shifts have cracked something open. In either case, the moral anxieties of this stage, the heightened self-consciousness, and the new capacity for abstract thought make intrusions more elaborate and compulsions more urgent.

Cultural and familial contexts also shape which themes surface most strongly. In some religious families, sexual thoughts outside of marriage may be viewed as shameful or corrupt, intensifying the adolescent's fear of immorality. In others, responsibility for others is emphasised above the self, so that any lapse feels like an unforgivable moral failure. More broadly, some cultures still interpret intrusive thoughts as signs of poor character or lack of self-control, which deepens shame and guilt.

To work in this storm is to hold both the developmental context and the individual history in mind. We must notice how the winds of puberty, personal and cultural identity formation, and moral questioning stir up old anxieties in new forms. And we must remember that these storms can be both destructive and transformative. In the chapters ahead, I will show how these shifting themes take on very different qualities depending on the adolescent's psychic position, from sealed retreat to persecutory dread to guilt and repair.

These developmental storms not only shape the content of obsessions and compulsions, they also expose the core tasks of adolescence itself.

Developmental Tasks and Vulnerabilities

Having traced how intrusive themes shift in adolescence, we now turn to the developmental tasks that dominate this period. These tasks are both achievements and vulnerabilities. They enlarge the adolescent's world but can also set the stage for OCD when earlier defences are reactivated and relied upon too rigidly.

Dependence, Autonomy, and the Search for Control

Adolescents push against parental boundaries while still relying on caregivers for safety and containment. This movement back and forth, the longing for independence and the pull toward dependence, is not a flaw in development but its heartbeat. It also heightens sensitivity to control, a theme that runs through much of OCD. Parents may be trusted companions one moment and dismissed the next. Criticising or devaluing them can make separation feel safer for a time, but it often stirs guilt and anxiety later. I often see how these tensions find their way into symptom life. Intrusive thoughts about harming parents, compulsions to protect or atone, rituals that try to keep love intact while pushing it away.

In clinical work, these dynamics rarely stay abstract. They show up in tone, timing, and in the therapeutic relationship itself. One week an adolescent may experience me as a useful companion in thinking; the next I am dismissed as irrelevant, as though all progress has evaporated. With OCD, this oscillation can be especially stark. A young person may leave a session confident and energised to attempt an exposure exercise, only to return the following week insisting the compulsion 'wasn't really so bad after all' and is not worth resisting. Progress lurches forward and backward in rhythm with the developmental storm of autonomy and dependence.

For the clinician, the task is to tolerate this volatility without rushing to stabilise it, recognising that the conflict between autonomy and dependence is being replayed in the therapeutic relationship itself. In some ways, these struggles repeat the early negotiation between dependence and separation that first unfolded in infancy, now restaged in a new and more complex register. Parents too can find themselves pulled between extremes: wanting to protect their child from distress yet feeling pushed away when they try. Their own anxieties about letting go can quietly reinforce the very cycles of reassurance the adolescent depends on. In this way, the struggle for independence becomes both a developmental milestone and fertile ground for obsessive doubt.

If we think about compulsions more broadly, they are often an attempt to regain a sense of control or certainty over an imagined outcome. Regardless of the specific content, young people will often say things like 'it just feels safer', 'just to be sure', or 'I can't handle not knowing'. If we zoom out from the symptom and place it within the wider context of adolescent development, this makes deep sense. Adolescence is, by its nature, a time when much feels beyond one's control.

In childhood, there is at least some predictability: the same teachers, familiar classrooms, regular routines, and friendships that tend to stay put. By adolescence, this scaffolding begins to loosen. Secondary school brings shifting peer groups, academic pressure, and an expanding social world that changes by the week. What was once stable becomes uncertain. Autonomy itself is both thrilling and terrifying because it carries genuine unpredictability.

Holding that tension is no small task. It asks the adolescent to tolerate both excitement and fear, to accept freedom without guarantee. In this light, OCD can be understood as a compromise formation, a psychic attempt to manage the chaos of emerging independence by creating artificial certainty. The compulsion becomes a small island of control in a sea of change.

As the body changes and sexuality becomes more tangible, thoughts themselves acquire new power. Feelings once safely contained in play or imagination now carry physical and moral weight, and the mind's struggle to master this awakening can make intrusive thoughts feel especially dangerous or taboo. This leads naturally to the next developmental task of adolescence: negotiating sexual and aggressive impulses.

Sexual and Aggressive Impulses

If autonomy tests the adolescent's tie to caregivers, sexuality and aggression test the adolescent's tie to their own body and the complicated feelings that come with it. Puberty transforms impulses that once felt harmless in childhood into forces that now carry a very different weight as the body changes shape and tone. Muscles form, voices deepen, height shoots up, and anger now arrives in a body that feels altered and powerful.

One young man told me, 'I'd never hurt my mum, but I'm worried that if I get angry, I may accidentally harm her. I just feel so angry for no reason.' His words captured something I have heard in many forms: a fear of the body's new potential, as though impulses that once passed through a smaller, lighter frame could now break out and cause real damage. These realisations are ordinary enough, but in some young people the fear that they might accidentally harm someone they love hardens into violent obsessions or compulsions to protect.

The developing body, with its new capacities for strength, speed. and sexual expression, can feel unpredictable, even alien. A growth spurt that arrives too fast, or the sudden awareness of being looked at or admired, can turn a source of pride into unease. The adolescent becomes frightened of their own body, not in a psychotic sense, but as if it were a creature with a will of its own. The wish to control this unpredictability, to manage the surge of physical power or desire, can easily translate into the language of compulsion. In OCD, this becomes a symbolic attempt to restrain impulses that feel both thrilling and dangerous.

Sexual impulses can be equally unsettling. New sensations and fantasies awaken at a pace the mind can barely keep up with. What once belonged safely to imagination becomes an actual possibility. A girl who once pushed a doll in a pram may suddenly realise she is physically capable of conceiving and carrying a child. This new agency can feel both surreal and frightening, and intrusive sexual thoughts often seize upon that shock. Obsessions with contamination, purity, or orientation are not random misfirings of the mind but symbolic ways of managing impulses that feel too powerful to be owned directly.

I recall a 14-year-old girl tormented by the thought that she might be pregnant despite never having had sexual contact. Each time she felt a bodily sensation – a stomach ache, a missed period – it became proof in her mind. Rational explanations offered no comfort. What terrified her was not the biological impossibility but the dawning sense that her body carried a power she could not fully control. For her, OCD fastened onto the confusion between fantasy and physical possibility, magnifying it into catastrophe. Here, sexual and aggressive impulses become the raw material for intrusive fear, with compulsions functioning as fragile attempts at containment.

Cognitive Shifts

The arrival of abstract thinking is one of adolescence's great achievements, yet it also opens new territory for OCD. Abstract thought allows young people to imagine scenarios, test possibilities in their minds, and reflect on themselves in ways that were not possible in childhood. For some, this brings freedom, but for others it becomes a trap, fuelling endless loops of doubt.

Many adolescents with OCD describe getting caught in spirals of existential questioning: 'What if none of this is real? What if my whole life is a dream?' For some, such questions are part of healthy exploration, a sign that the mind is stretching into new dimensions. For others, however, the same capacity feeds pathological doubt. One boy told me, 'If I can imagine the world ending, then maybe it actually could.' What should be a liberating skill, the ability to step outside the immediate and consider alternatives, becomes instead a prison of uncertainty and fear.

Here, magical thinking returns in subtle disguise. The adolescent knows their rituals are irrational, yet the feeling insists otherwise. The logic of omnipotence survives in cognitive form: if a thought can imagine it, perhaps it can make it happen. Developmental growth and obsessive doubt become entwined, making it hard to see where normal questioning ends and pathological obsession begins.

I have listened to young people ask, with tears in their eyes, whether their family is real, or whether they might be living in a simulation. For them, existential thought is not gentle curiosity but torment. What should be an expansion of mind becomes a collapse into rumination, each new idea feeding doubt rather than discovery. In such cases, cognitive development becomes the very stage on which OCD rehearses its most corrosive forms of uncertainty.

Peer and Social Pressures

If abstract thought stretches the adolescent's mind, peer culture stretches their sense of self. In adolescence, identity becomes bound up with peer approval. I often notice how young people edit what they share with me depending on whether they think it sounds 'too weird' or 'too babyish'. Shame and secrecy can silence them just when symptoms are most intense. Friends sometimes try to help but end up strengthening the rituals. I remember one girl whose friends kindly agreed to let her tap her right elbow against theirs if it had brushed the left side, a way of undoing bad luck. They were supporting her, but in doing so they were also reinforcing the compulsion.

The same dynamic now plays out online. Adolescents watch one another on TikTok or Instagram, comparing not only how they look but also how they speak about their own mental health. Some find relief in discovering others with OCD. Others feel trapped by the pressure to present their struggles as quirky or even admirable. I have heard young people say, 'It's nice to know I'm not alone,' followed by, 'But I don't feel like that kind of OCD person.' The result is that compulsions can become folded into peer culture, hidden in plain sight. In the therapy room this often shows up as hesitation: the young person checking my reaction, as if to see whether I will collude like a peer or hold the ritual at a different level.

I recall a boy who told me that he would post late at night about his OCD struggles and then lie awake scrolling, counting how many 'likes' the post received. Each notification gave him a brief lift, but when the numbers dipped or a friend did not comment, he became flooded with doubt: maybe they don't believe me, maybe I'm faking this, maybe I don't really have OCD. What began as a bid for connection became another ritual of checking and reassurance, only this time enacted on a public stage. It showed me how easily the digital world can entangle itself with the private logic of OCD, turning what should be a lifeline into another cycle of doubt.

For many, peer culture both soothes and destabilises. The same friends who offer comfort can become mirrors for comparison. Their lives appear neater, lighter, untouched by the strange burden of compulsions. And so, OCD here feeds on the adolescent hunger for belonging, transforming the social world into a stage for obsession and compulsion alike.

The Body and Visibility

If peers extend the adolescent's world outward, the body becomes the unavoidable ground on which that world is lived. One of the most striking parts of adolescence is how suddenly the body feels on display. Changes in shape, skin, voice, or hair seem to carry a spotlight of their own. Some young people meet this with bravado, others with embarrassment, shame, or withdrawal. In my consulting room I often see hoodies pulled tight, sleeves covering hands, faces half hidden. It is as if the adolescent is trying to undo the fact of being seen.

Over the years, I have relied on low lighting in the consulting room, avoiding the harsh overhead glare of white lights. Instead, I use a lamp that gives off a softer, warmer glow. This is a simple ergonomic choice, but I have often observed adolescents relax a little when they are not exposed to the unforgiving brightness that highlights every feature of their face and skin. Such small details remind me that the adolescent body is not only a biological fact but also a psychic stage, where visibility itself can feel dangerous.

This sense of exposure is not only about appearance but about power. Feminist psychoanalytic writers have long noted how the developing female body is often met with intrusive attention and loss of privacy. I have worked with girls who felt that even walking to school was a gauntlet of being watched, appraised, or judged. Boys too can feel scrutinised. Erections in public, voice cracks in class, or the first signs of facial hair bring their own dread of humiliation. These moments are rarely spoken of, yet they saturate the adolescent atmosphere.

Some psychoanalytic theorists, especially Meltzer in his discussions of claustrum phenomena, invite us to consider how emerging bodily boundaries carry unconscious significance and may generate confusion (Laufer & Laufer, 1984). In adolescence, when reproductive capacity becomes real, these confusions resurface with particular intensity. I remember a young woman describing the shock of realising she could now conceive a child. What once was play, pushing a doll in a pram, had become a biological possibility, and the thought filled her with dread. Intrusive sexual and pregnancy obsessions often fasten on this new awareness, blurring the boundary between possibility and fantasy.

For some, compulsions act like symbolic shields. A girl may wash repeatedly, as if cleansing away the imagined stain of being looked at. A boy may count or check, as if rituals could hold back the shame of his body's unpredictability. One young person told me that keeping their hoodie up in every session 'kept the thoughts inside'. It was not simply about comfort but about containment, as if fabric itself could protect against being seen and known too deeply. In this way, the body becomes both stage and prison. The same changes that mark growth and possibility can also be lived as exposure and danger. Compulsions do not erase this conflict, but they offer adolescents a sense, however temporary, of being shielded from view.

When Early Shadows Return

If adolescence brings new challenges, it also reawakens old ones. Rituals often fade in latency, when impulses quieten and the child seems settled, but in adolescence the same themes return with symbolic force. This is not regression in any trivial sense but the mind drawing again on older solutions under new pressures. What was once kept at bay in latency now reappears with urgency, as if the predictability of that period has been shattered.

As explored earlier, rituals from childhood often reappear in adolescence with new symbolic intensity, especially under pressure from bodily change and moral conflict.

Parents may remember these habits with a kind of nostalgia, but the adolescent experiences them with dread. The same behaviour that once looked quirky or even sweet is now felt as unbearable responsibility. Under the pressure of bodily change, shifting peer allegiances, and moral self-scrutiny, these earlier strategies are reactivated and reshaped.

Developmental research shows that ritualistic routines increase in toddlerhood and preschool years, then lessen during latency, with most youngsters showing a marked decline by middle childhood (Evans et al., 1997; Zohar & Felz, 2001). A small subgroup, however, continues to display pronounced "just right" tendencies into later childhood (De Caluwé et al., 2020). Across developmental and neurobiological studies, one sees a recurring theme: children whose early rituals harden rather than fade often grow more anxious, sometimes tipping into obsessive-compulsive habits later on (Liu & Fan, 2023; Becker et al., 2023). Together, these studies remind us that ritual is not simply a developmental phase but, in some children, a sign of enduring vulnerability.

From a psychodynamic perspective, the reappearance of familiar rituals in adolescence signals a return of earlier challenges in a more symbolically charged register. As young people struggle again with separation and autonomy, older fears about safety, loss, and responsibility are reactivated. Concerns about dirt become moral contamination, counting rituals ward off imagined disasters, and checking behaviours defend against intrusive aggressive or sexual impulses. Behaviours that once organised a toddler's world can foreshadow more enduring struggles when they persist beyond their normative window.

I recall a boy of 15 whose parents described him as having been 'fussy' about bedtime since he was small. As a child, he insisted on a fixed sequence: curtains drawn, door checked, duvet smoothed three times. Back then it looked like routine, a way of settling to sleep. In adolescence it returned with a new edge. He now checked the door repeatedly, not to be sure it was shut but to prevent the possibility of an intruder killing his family while they slept. He confessed to lying awake for hours, straining to remember whether the latch had clicked, replaying the sound in his head until dawn. What his parents had once regarded as a harmless quirk had re-emerged as an exhausting, catastrophic ritual, transformed by the pressures of adolescence into something frightening and uncontainable.

For clinicians, these 'early shadows' are crucial. They reveal both the child's earlier strategies for managing unmanageable feelings and the present-day pressures that have called them back into service. To overlook them is to miss the thread linking past to present in the adolescent's obsessive-compulsive story. These shadows do not simply repeat what has gone before. In adolescence they are reshaped, taking on new symbolic charge once the young person can imagine futures, moral consequences, and catastrophic outcomes. It is to this transformation of meaning that I now turn.

The Adolescent Mind and the Transformation of OCD Themes

In adolescence, thinking itself is transformed. Young people can imagine futures both pleasurable and disastrous, weigh moral consequences, and reflect on identity in ways that were not possible in childhood. Compulsions that once guarded against concrete dangers are now reinterpreted through this new lens: contamination becomes corruption, checking doors becomes checking feelings, counting shifts from warding off bad luck to ensuring that nothing terrible happens within the self. What matters is not only the change in content but the change in meaning.

Here, cognitive behavioural therapy (CBT), as explored further in Chapter 6, can be invaluable in unearthing meaning. CBT for OCD often highlights that it is the personal meaning given to an intrusive thought that sparks anxiety and in turn drives the compulsion. Even within a cognitive frame, it remains vital to pause and explore what a thought signifies to the young person, rather than rushing to neutralise or correct it. Yet this is not always straightforward. Adolescents can be highly guarded and defended, and uncovering what lies beneath a thought or image can feel like trying to approach something hidden behind thick glass. Intrusions are no longer fleeting fears; they are lived as predictions about the self: 'Someone will die if I do not do this tapping ritual,' or, 'What if something awful happens because of me?' Fears about failing to complete rituals, or about the imagined consequences of a lapse, are common throughout my clinical experience.

I often hear adolescents describe their thoughts as if they have uncovered a hidden truth. 'Maybe this means I'm dangerous,' or, 'What if this shows who I really am?' The thought is not experienced as passing but as revelation. Sitting with them, I sometimes feel the weight of that conviction pressing into the room, as though doubt itself has become a solid object between us.

There is often an instinctive pull to reassure them that they are not what they fear, but such verbal reassurance can model the idea that these thoughts are too unbearable to think about and must be corrected. Instead, one has to hold the line and show that it is possible to sit with uncertainty.

The more vivid their imagination, the more persuasive the obsession becomes. I have often noticed, perhaps coincidentally, perhaps reflecting a genuine connection, that those who are more creative through writing, art, or music tend to struggle more intensely. It is as though they are the architects of their own minds, capable of designing not only inspiring ideas but also intricate, tortuous structures of how they believe things must be. Their creativity, which elsewhere gives shape to expression and identity, here turns inward, constructing elaborate systems of mental control.

In my experience, this is where interventions like CBT can reach their limit. When a young person's body has created such deep structures of control, it becomes extraordinarily difficult to disassemble them through further cognitive methods alone. This doubleness, knowing a thought is irrational yet experiencing it as profoundly true, is one of the most destabilising qualities of adolescence. A 13-year-old may insist they know their thought cannot cause harm, while in the same breath confess that not repeating a phrase would feel tantamount to killing a sibling. In the consulting room, I too become caught in this doubleness. In one session I may be pulled to collude with the certainty of the fear, as though my agreement could secure them against catastrophe. In the next, I may be treated as naive for failing to grasp the thought's power. To sit in this push and pull without resorting to premature reassurance is one of the hardest disciplines of working with OCD in adolescence. It demands a quiet steadiness, a refusal to join either side of the conflict too quickly, allowing something of the adolescent's divided experience to be felt and thought about rather than acted upon.

Parents often find this transformation equally bewildering. They remember the harmless rituals of childhood, only to see them return in darker, more elaborate form. One father said to me, 'I thought she'd grown out of all that. Now it feels like it's come back but more distressing for her.' What he sensed was not only the return of ritual but its new symbolic charge. Attempts to treat these behaviours as they did years earlier, with distraction, reassurance, or gentle coaxing, rarely touch the depth of dread the adolescent now feels. Parents may describe feeling helpless, as though their usual instincts to comfort have been short-circuited. Some oscillate between irritation and fear, torn between wanting to challenge the rituals and fearing the emotional collapse that might follow.

For the young person, rituals that once anchored bedtime or transitions now seem to carry life-or-death consequences. Compulsions become fragile protections against unbearable uncertainty, while intrusive thoughts are lived as dangerous revelations of identity. The moral imagination that is opening up in adolescence the new capacity to think about guilt, responsibility, and consequence becomes drawn into the service of obsession. Childhood shadows return, but refracted through new bodily realities, moral consciousness, and the fragile work of identity that makes adolescence such a precarious time. To work with OCD in adolescence is to sit in storms that are both familiar and strange. The same behaviours reappear, but their meaning is transformed. What once seemed like ritual now functions as a private language of survival. In the chapters that follow, I turn to the psychic positions through which these storms take shape, beginning with the claustral states that some young people retreat into when the turbulence of thought and feeling becomes overwhelming.

Conclusion: Holding the Storm

Adolescence reanimates the residues of childhood OCD but does not leave them unchanged. Earlier rituals and themes return with new force, reshaped by bodily growth, sexuality, and moral awakening. What once soothed becomes catastrophic, what once anchored becomes imprisoning.

For clinicians, the task is to hold this doubleness in mind, to recognise continuity without collapsing it into mere repetition, and to grasp transformation without forgetting its developmental roots. The storm of adolescence is not only in the adolescent's mind but also in the therapeutic relationship, where certainty and doubt, closeness and withdrawal, are replayed with unsettling force.

In this chapter, I have shown how childhood shadows return in adolescence, refracted through new bodily realities and symbolic intensities. What strikes me most, sitting with these storms, is that the thought is rarely the true beginning. Rituals may shift with puberty, but what drives them is the weight of feeling shame, rage, guilt, desire too much to hold directly. Before the thought comes the feeling. It is to there, in the rawness of affect that precedes the intrusion, that the next chapter turns.

References

Anderson, R., & Dartington, A. (Eds.). (1998). *Facing it out: Clinical perspectives on adolescent disturbance.* London and New York: Routledge. doi:10.4324/9780429474514.

Becker, H., Liu, Y., Hanna, G. L., Fitzgerald, K., Rosso, I. M., & March, J. S. (2023). Error-related brain activity associated with obsessive–compulsive symptoms in youth. *Brain and Behavior*, 13(4), e2941. doi:10.1002/brb3.2941.

Bion, W. R. (1970). *Attention and interpretation.* London: Tavistock Publications.

De Caluwé, E., Vergauwe, J., Decuyper, M., Bogaerts, S., Rettew, D. C., & De Clercq, B. (2020). The relation between normative rituals/routines and obsessive-compulsive symptoms at a young age: A systematic review. *Developmental Review*, 56, article 100913. doi:10.1016/j.dr.2020.100913.

Evans, D. W., Leckman, J. F., Carter, A., Reznick, J. S., Henshaw, D., King, R. A., & Pauls, D. (1997). Ritual, habit, and perfectionism: The prevalence and development of compulsive-like behavior in normal young children. *Child Development*, 68(1), 58–68. doi:10.1111/j.1467-8624.1997.tb01925.x.

Freud, A. (1958). Adolescence. *The Psychoanalytic Study of the Child*, 13, 255–278. doi:10.1080/00797308.1958.11823182.

Freud, A. (1937/1968). *The ego and the mechanisms of defence* (C. Baines, Trans., rev. ed.). London: Hogarth Press. (Original work published 1936.)

Freud, S. (1905/1953). Three essays on the theory of sexuality. In J. Strachey (Ed. & Trans.), *The standard edition of the complete psychological works of Sigmund Freud* (Vol. VII, pp. 123–246). London: Hogarth Press.

Johnson, S. B., Blum, R. W., & Giedd, J. N. (2009). Adolescent maturity and the brain: The promise and pitfalls of neuroscience research in adolescent health. *Journal of Adolescent Health*, 45(3), 216–221. doi:10.1016/j.jadohealth.2009.05.016.

Laufer, M., & Laufer, M. E. (1984). *Adolescence and developmental breakdown.* London: Hogarth Press. doi:10.4324/9780429471612.

Liu, X., & Fan, Q. (2023). Early identification and intervention in pediatric obsessive-compulsive disorder. *Brain Sciences*, 13(3), article 399. doi:10.3390/brainsci13030399.

Meltzer, D., & Harris, M. (1986). *Adolescence: Talks and papers.* Paris: Clunie Press.

Mercurio, E., García-López, E., Morales-Quintero, L. A., Llamas, N. E., Marinaro, J. Á., & Muñoz, J. M. (2020). Adolescent brain development and progressive legal responsibility in the Latin American context. *Frontiers in Psychology*, 11, article 627. doi:10.3389/fpsyg.2020.00627.

Midgley, N., Mortimer, R., Cirasola, A., Batra, P., & Kennedy, E. (2021). The evidence-base for psychodynamic psychotherapy with children and adolescents: A narrative synthesis. *Frontiers in Psychology*, 12, article 662671. doi:10.3389/fpsyg.2021.662671.

Oliveira, J. T., Ribeiro, A. P., & Gonçalves, M. M. (2020). Ambivalence in psychotherapy questionnaire: Development and validation studies. *Clinical Psychology & Psychotherapy*, 27 (5), 727–735. doi:10.1002/cpp.2457.

Sikand, M., & Bhola, P. (2024). Push and pull: Role of therapist mentalizing in navigating therapeutic distance. *Indian Journal of Psychological Medicine*, 46(3), doi:10.1177/02537176241231930.

Winnicott, D. W. (1963). Adolescence: Struggling through the doldrums. In L. Caldwell & H. T. Robinson (Eds.), *The collected works of D. W. Winnicott: Volume 6, 1960–1963* (pp. 187–196). Oxford: Oxford University Press. doi:10.1093/med:psych/9780190271381.003.0027.

Zohar, A. H., & Felz, L. (2001). Ritualistic behavior in young children. *Journal of Abnormal Child Psychology*, 29(2), 121–128. doi:10.1023/A:1005231912747.

Before the Thought, the Feeling

Before the thought, the feeling. It is a simple phrase, but in clinic it can be difficult to see and think about. By the time a young person arrives at our door, the thought has usually taken over – loud, intrusive, and terrifying. The feeling that birthed it lies buried underneath, silent but alive. This chapter begins there, in that moment just before the mind splits experience into thought and defence.

She is 15 years old and has barely spoken during the first two sessions. Her responses are closed off, even to neutral and open-ended questions. I sense she feels the need to communicate quickly and succinctly, so that nothing slips out which might terrify her, or me. On the third session she looks up suddenly and blurts, 'I keep thinking I might stab my best friend. I don't want to. But I can't stop it.' She looks horrified. She hides her face in her sleeves, pulls up her hoody, and folds her hands tightly into her palms. The communication is laced with fear and urgency. Logically I know what this is – intrusive thoughts – yet it stirs urgency in me, a desire to act and respond. In that moment, however, what she needs is not an abstract lecture about the normality of intrusive thoughts or misfiring brain circuits. She needs someone to stay with the rawness of her fear, to recognise that beneath the content of the thought lies a feeling she cannot yet put into words.

This is not easy. In moments like this, one's qualifications, publications, even years of clinical experience can feel strangely inadequate. They sit there, silent and polished, offering little in the face of something so raw. Faced with such intensity, it's easy to feel as though you have nothing of substance to offer beyond hollow reassurance. The mind reaches for something useful, something clever or calming to say, but she is not asking for cleverness. She is asking if her terror can be borne.

This encounter captures the central premise of this chapter: that the thought itself is rarely the true beginning. Before we can map its mechanics, we must attend to the feeling that gives it force. Only then do theories of mind and brain begin to make sense of what happens in the room.

Many books on OCD begin with the mechanics of thoughts, how they arise, how they go wrong, how they repeat. This chapter starts elsewhere. It

DOI: 10.4324/9781003729716-5

begins with emotion. Bion once wrote that 'reason is emotion's slave and exists to rationalise emotional experience' (1970, p. 22). Feelings come first. Thoughts, including intrusive ones, often follow as attempts to symbolise or manage those feelings. The thought may look like the problem, but it is the emotional undercurrent that gives it its charge. As powerful and dominant as this charge is, it is often just outside the conscious awareness of the person experiencing the intrusive thought.

Neuroscience echoes this. As LeDoux (1996) demonstrated, emotional processing often begins along a rapid subcortical pathway, with the amygdala responding before higher cortical regions weave meaning; a physiological echo of how, psychically, feeling precedes though. Only afterward does the Default Mode Network (Raichle, 2015), the brain's narrative system, weave the feeling into a story. By the time a young person is tormented by an intrusive image, the emotional spark has already fired. The thought is not the starting point, but the aftershock. This aftershock is often followed by behaviours that attempt to neutralise it, the compulsions.

Seen in this way, intrusive thoughts are not random misfires but emotional residues, shaped into symbols the young person cannot yet decode. To understand them, we have to listen not only to what is thought, but to what was felt just before the thought arrived. That is rarely simple. When I try to explore this with adolescents, they often meet me with blankness: 'I wasn't feeling anything,' or, 'I was fine,' or the more common, 'Nothing, I don't think.' I have learned over time that it is often more useful not to press too soon. In the early stages of therapy, curiosity about the feeling behind the thought can feel intrusive or exposing. It is usually wiser to let the relationship do some of the work first, to create enough safety for those feelings to surface in their own time.

It is with this lens, before the thought, the feeling, that I now turn to a case example. The story of Adam illustrates how intrusive thoughts, however violent they appear, are stitched to deeper emotional truths.

The Story Behind the Thought

Every intrusive thought that is followed by a compulsion carries a story underneath. The thought is rarely random, it is the surface form of something emotional and unarticulated pressing for recognition. Over the years, many ideas have been put forward by psychoanalytic and non-psychoanalytic writers to explain this process. While it is beyond the scope of this book to critically appraise them all, I will offer a selective survey of those concepts that remain influential in contemporary clinical thinking. To do this, I will stay close to an actual clinical case involving a boy named Adam.

Intrusive thoughts do not emerge in a vacuum. They are stitched to feelings, often hidden at first glance. Consider Adam, aged 13. He arrives in therapy consumed by images of harming his younger brother. He avoids him at the dinner table, retreats from games, and spends long nights scanning his own mind for danger. On the surface, it looks like a fear of violence. But beneath it, something quieter is at work.

As our sessions unfold, a deeper picture emerges. Adam feels invisible. His sibling draws praise while he sits in the shadows. Jealousy simmers, raw and unspoken, but unacceptable within his moral code. Raised to believe that good brothers love and protect, even the hint of resentment threatens his identity. The intrusive thought, 'What if I hurt him?' is not random. It is the distorted symbol of a feeling Adam cannot consciously allow. The nightly scanning is the compulsion, his desperate ritual to prove he remains safe, that his love is intact, that nothing violent lurks within.

Bion (1962) described such moments as collisions between preconceptions, the unconscious expectation of being the 'good brother', and intrusive truths, jealousy, and shame. When they fuse, they generate something vivid and unbearable, a thought that feels real, not symbolic. This is why intrusive thoughts carry such power. They do not announce themselves as fictions, they arrive as revelations.

Other intrusive thoughts can be understood in this way too. A contamination fear may be the collision of an unconscious wish to remain pure with a hidden anger that feels dirty or spoiling, a blasphemous image may be the collision of a deep wish to belong spiritually with an intrusive doubt or resentment toward authority. If we translated this into cognitive behavioural therapy (CBT) language, we might end up speaking of 'core beliefs'. But Bion's conception runs at another level altogether, less about conscious belief, more about the unconscious expectation that shapes whether a thought strikes as unbearable.

Adam's story shows us how intrusive thoughts can crystallise disowned feelings. But sometimes, the issue is not simply disowned it is undeveloped altogether. This brings us to Christopher Bollas's idea of the unthought known.

The Unthought Known

Christopher Bollas, a British psychoanalyst writing in the late 1980s, named something that many clinicians already sensed: the unthought known (1987). This is experiences that were never fully put into words but settled into the psyche all the same. They live on as moods, family roles, or the felt tone of a household. They are not remembered; they are carried. When certain emotional states arise, these unspoken truths press forward, not as stories but as sensations, fears, or thoughts that do not seem to fit. From a contemporary perspective, we might recognise this as the body keeping score, traces of experience carried in implicit memory that speak without words.

I want to pause here, because, although this may sound like a digression, it matters. Trauma research has shown that what cannot be thought in infancy is often carried somatically. I am reminded of a 16-year-old I worked with using eye movement desensitisation and reprocessing (EMDR) after a mugging. As he described his fear, he spoke of sharp, burning pain shooting through his back, and as he spoke the sensation returned. It later emerged that in his first week of life there had been a medical error during a lumbar puncture. He knew nothing of this, and his family had never spoken of it, yet his body seemed to remember. This is not an isolated finding but something documented repeatedly in the trauma field (van der Kolk, 2014; Schore, 2003).

Writers in other disciplines have noticed the same pattern. Systemic therapists speak of family scripts, expectations carried quietly across generations. Cognitive scientists describe implicit memory and bias, the traces of experience that shape behaviour without our awareness. The terms differ, but the reality is familiar: not all knowledge is consciously thinkable, yet it still shapes how we live and feel.

This is why I can have patience when an adolescent repeatedly says, 'I don't know.' It is not always resistance or lack of effort, although at times it can be that too. More often, it is because they genuinely do not know. Something is being felt or lived that has not yet reached words. My task is to stay close to that gap until language begins to emerge.

For Adam, the idea that he must always be the protector was never spoken aloud, yet it lived in him all the same. The thought of harming his brother threatened that hidden identity. The intrusive thought was not a prophecy; it was a rupture, a break between who he believed he should be and what he unconsciously felt. His nightly scanning rituals were his way of repairing that break, searching for reassurance that he remained safe and intact as the good brother he needed to be.

A similar pattern appeared in a girl who scrubbed her hands until they bled, convinced she was dirty inside. In her family, emotions were never spoken, yet the air was thick with unacknowledged anger. What pressed forward in her rituals was not a fear of germs but the weight of aggression she could not own. My understanding of her experience, and what gradually became our shared understanding, was that her handwashing was her way of scrubbing at feelings that had no name.

A boy raised in a devout household was tormented by sudden images of insulting God during prayer or urinating on the cross. He loved his faith and feared losing it. Nothing in his conscious mind wished to rebel, yet beneath the surface lay frustration and doubt that had no room for expression. Again, what we came to understand together was that these thoughts were not evidence of disbelief but the pressure of unspoken ambivalence. The intrusive images forced into consciousness what could not be expressed directly.

Therapeutically, this requires more than reassurance. It calls for translation. The task is to help the young person find words for what they could not think before. The aim is not to drive the thought away but to integrate the feeling that fuels it, so that the terror of the image or ritual gives way to understanding the emotion beneath.

If the unthought known helps us grasp what is silently carried within, projective identification shows us what happens when those unspoken feelings are pushed outward, only to return as something alien.

Projective Identification

Some intrusive thoughts feel so alien that the young person insists they could not have come from within. 'It is like the thought was put into my head,' one adolescent told me. Another said, 'I feel like my thoughts are not my own anymore. I know that sounds crazy, and I know obviously they are mine, but it's so hard to explain.'

This strangeness can be illuminated by a core psychoanalytic idea: projective identification (Klein, 1946; Bion, 1962). The idea rests on the notion that unwanted feelings are pushed outward and then experienced as if they live elsewhere, in another person or in some foreign place.

Before we go further, it is important to clarify how I am using the term. Projective identification is a universal concept in psychotherapy, but it has been written about in different ways across traditions (Waska, 2021; Spillius & O'Shaughnessy, 2012). When I refer to it, I am thinking within a two-person psychology: the projector, in this case the adolescent, has a feeling that is unbearable and pushes it outward onto another person, often the clinician. If the clinician begins to literally feel that feeling and identify with it, they have entered the process of projective identification.

Why does this matter? If I arrive in a calm state of mind and soon find myself heavy with hopelessness, helplessness, or some other feeling that seems foreign to me, I need to pause. If I fail to recognise this as an identification with a projected feeling, I risk losing my own emotional footing. My lack of optimism may seep into the room, leaving both of us trapped in the same hopelessness.

To make this more concrete, I think of moments in the consulting room when I have suddenly felt sad or oddly helpless even as the adolescent opposite me insisted everything was fine. Their sadness had been pushed into me. My task was to recognise that the feeling was not originally mine and to return it in a form that could be thought about: 'As you say everything is fine, I notice I feel quite sad inside, almost helpless. Is that a feeling you've ever had?' This is not a trick or clever interpretation; it is an attempt to give shape to what was unspoken, to help the young person take it back in a way that can be thought about.

Of course, I can appreciate that colleagues who work in a more active or structured way may not give such feelings much credit, or may dismiss them as countertransference. That may sometimes be true. But projection and projective identification are happening all the time, shaping the atmosphere of the room whether we notice them or not.

With intrusive thoughts, the projection can circle back in distorted form, creating the sense of an alien intruder in the mind. A girl who feared she might poison her parents' food described the image as though it had been planted from outside. Over time, it became clearer that what pressed beneath was resentment at being constantly corrected and criticised at home. The mind had cast out what it could not bear, only for it to return as a persecutory thought.

I have seen the same process in contamination fears. A young person may feel something frightening inside them – disgust, shame, or embarrassment – that cannot be owned. These feelings get projected onto a door handle, which suddenly seems dangerous and dirty. The adolescent avoids the handle, or performs elaborate cleansing rituals after touching it, in a desperate attempt to keep those feelings at a distance. My understanding, and what can become our shared understanding, is that the ritual is less about germs than about managing emotions that feel too unsafe to recognise as their own.

This is also where cognitive behavioural models can be useful. The cycle of projection and avoidance easily becomes self-reinforcing, and CBT helps to map this sequence of thoughts, feelings, and behaviours as responses to perceived threat. The two approaches do not cancel one another out but can complement each other, each offering a different way into the same emotional circuit.

Projective identification shows how unbearable feelings can be pushed outward and then return as something alien or foreign, as though planted from outside. Yet there are other situations where the feeling is not projected but lies dormant, never symbolised in the first place. In these moments the anxiety in the room can feel less like a specific intrusion and more like a background dread, as though something catastrophic has already happened but cannot be spoken. It is here that Winnicott's idea of the fear of breakdown becomes especially relevant.

Winnicott: Fear of Breakdown (1974)

Winnicott added yet another layer with his idea of the fear of breakdown (1974). For him, the terror was not of some future catastrophe that adolescents bring into the consulting room when they talk about their anxiety but of a collapse that had already been lived but never emotionally processed. The adolescent's intrusive thought can be seen from this perspective: not a prediction of danger, but the disguised return of an earlier, unthinkable anxiety that lacked containment at the time. What re-emerges is not new, but something that was never fully experienced.

This resonates with me strongly in work with a 13-year-old who had a very challenging start to life. After a medical emergency at home, she spent her first four months in an incubator. In the consulting room it always felt as though she was 'fighting for her life'. Yet outwardly her world was functioning well; she attended school, had friendships, and could acknowledge her own progress. Still, there was a constant sense of something terrifying about to happen, a dread she could never quite name. Over the months of working together, we were able to speak about those early experiences. Although no conscious memory could be born, linking her present fears to the intensity of those beginnings helped us both to understand the depth of what she carried.

Repression offers yet another pathway by which feelings make their disguised return. To understand how, we turn now to Freud's enduring account.

Return of the Repressed

Freud (1915) described another process that still feels strikingly relevant: repression. When an unacceptable impulse or emotion is pushed from awareness, it does not disappear. It returns in disguise, often distorted and intensified. For Adam, the jealousy and guilt he could not acknowledge returned as violent images that terrified him. The mind was not punishing him, it was trying in the only way it could to show what had not been felt. I am also reminded of a young woman who dropped a tin of tomatoes in a supermarket. It clattered to the floor with little consequence, no one paid much attention, and the tin was undamaged. Yet she collapsed in tears, appearing destroyed by the event. Objectively, her reaction seemed disproportionate, but in reality, she had been pushing feelings away all day. The small, innocuous accident opened the floodgates, and everything repressed rushed out at once. What looked like an overreaction was in fact the disguised return of what had been held down.

I have seen this process in other forms too. A boy raised in a deeply religious household described relentless blasphemous images. What returned in his mind was not an attack on God, but his repressed anger at being silenced within the family. Another adolescent came fearful of contamination. In our work together it became clearer that she was not only warding off germs, but also struggling with disowned feelings of disgust about her own emerging sexuality, feelings she could not yet allow into awareness.

Repression works as a defensive act, protecting a young person from being overwhelmed by inner conflict in the short term. But what is repressed does not vanish. It comes back symbolically, often more disturbing precisely because its origin is hidden. This is why I so often find that intrusive thoughts, however alien they appear, are really disguised messengers of feelings that cannot yet be thought directly.

It is worth stressing that Freud's idea of repression is often misunderstood. I sometimes hear people assume that if someone has violent thoughts toward a parent or sibling, then somewhere deep down they must want to act on them. This is a gross misreading. While negative feelings toward loved ones are inevitable in every family, the intrusive thought is not a direct wish to harm. In my experience, it is the mind's attempt to give shape to conflict and ambivalence that cannot be faced in plain form.

Adolescence makes this especially vivid. Sexual and aggressive drives surge, the moral conscience sharpens, and the adolescent becomes more acutely aware of what feels taboo. What cannot be faced openly may be forced out of mind, only to return as an image, a compulsion, or a dread that feels unexplainable. Freud's century-old observation remains relevant here. Repression is not the end of a feeling, but the beginning of its disguised return.

So far, we have seen that intrusive thoughts may emerge from collisions of expectation, as outlined by Bion; from unformulated residues, as reflected by Bollas; from projected disowning, a process explored by both Klein and Bion; or from disguised returns, first articulated by Freud. But what happens when the very capacity to think about feelings falters altogether?

When Thinking Breaks Down

Fonagy and colleagues (2002) would describe Adam as struggling with mentalisation, the capacity to reflect on one's own and others' mental states. Without this capacity, emotional experiences remain raw, unprocessed, and confusing. Thoughts become fused with identity. If I think I might harm someone, it must mean I want to. There is no distance between thought and self.

An astute reader might ask how this differs from omnipotent thought, where thinking something is felt to make it so. The distinction, I believe, lies in the emotional position. Omnipotent thought belongs more to early infancy or psychotic states, where the boundary between internal and external is fluid and thoughts are experienced as causing events. What we often see in adolescents is something more fragile. It is not the belief that thought causes action, but the fear that thought defines self. The adolescent doesn't believe the thought will make something happen. Rather, they fear it reveals something shameful about who they already are.

This collapse in internal space is often what fuels the intensity of distress. Therapy, then, becomes a place where the thought can be observed rather than obeyed. Where the adolescent can begin to say, 'I had the thought,' instead of, 'I am the thought.'

This is similar in some ways to the cognitive behavioural idea of defusion, where the young person learns to say, 'I notice I'm having the thought that I'm a bad person,' rather than fusing entirely with the thought. But, in my experience, the shift is not just cognitive. The adolescent needs to feel the emotional truth of that distinction too.

I have often noticed that adolescents who struggle most with intrusive thoughts also find it difficult to take perspectives more broadly. They may struggle to imagine that others have different intentions, or to understand that feelings can exist without being acted upon. When emotional states are experienced as facts rather than experiences to reflect on, the result is a kind of psychic entrapment. A violent image becomes proof of being violent. A sexual thought becomes evidence of being perverse.

This is why therapeutic work that fosters mentalisation is so essential. Helping a young person pause and reflect creates just enough space to shift the equation. A clinician might say, 'You had the thought. What do you think the thought was trying to tell you about how you were feeling?' In doing so, we begin to turn the intrusive image back into an emotional signal, rather than a terrifying self-definition.

Sometimes this work is painstakingly slow. I remember one girl who said, 'If I think about my mum dying, it must mean I want it.' We spent weeks disentangling the thought from her sense of self. In time, we were able to see together that the thought usually appeared when she felt ignored at home, angry at her mother's inattention. Once she could hold that distinction, between the wish to be noticed and the fantasy of her mother's death, the thought began to loosen its grip.

When thinking breaks down, the adolescent cannot yet symbolise what they feel. Our task, as therapists, is to lend them our reflective function, our capacity to think about what is being felt and why, until they begin to build that capacity for themselves. In this way, therapy does not simply treat the thought. It helps build the ability to think.

This brings us back, with sharper focus, to the heart of the chapter's claim: before the thought, the feeling. If intrusive thoughts are emotional aftershocks, then the therapeutic task is not simply to weaken the thought but to help the adolescent recover the feeling beneath.

The bridges between psychoanalytic and cognitive behavioural models converge here: both ask us to trace not just the content of the thought but the life of the feeling underneath. Without this attention, therapy risks treating the echo while missing the cry that came before.

But What Was I Feeling First?

If, as we have seen, intrusive thoughts are often aftershocks of unprocessed feeling, then the question in the room becomes, what was the feeling first? If intrusive thoughts are emotional responses in disguise, one way to reduce their power is to identify the primary feeling underneath. But this is not simple work. Most adolescents come to therapy focused on the content of the thought and how it makes them feel, not on the emotional life beneath it. They say:

> I keep thinking I'll hurt someone.
> I can't stop thinking about that mistake.

What if I'm secretly evil?
What if I catch a disease?
What if I insult God in my head?

They rarely say:

I feel rejected.
I'm ashamed.
I wish I were more important at home.
I still feel dirty after being teased.
I'm afraid of letting my family down.

And why would they? They are in pain. They want the thought to stop. They are not here to write poetry about guilt or shame. What they need is someone who can stay with the thought long enough to sense what lies beneath it.

In practice, this often means tracking when the thoughts are loudest, what preceded them, and what emotional residue they carry. A fear of contamination might echo a moment of humiliation or disgust that was never spoken. A blasphemous thought might carry the weight of a moral fear that has not yet found words.

Therapy becomes the space where the clinician helps make that link. Not by rushing to reassure, but by creating enough safety, patience, and space for the feeling to surface. Slowly, the adolescent begins to glimpse that the thought is not a revelation of who they are, but a signal of what they have felt. In that small shift, something new becomes possible.

From a cognitive behavioural perspective, this work might begin with identifying the antecedent event, mapping how it triggered the thought, and exploring the meaning attached to it. This can be helpful, particularly when it highlights the role of interpretation and meaning. But if applied too narrowly, it can miss the emotional terrain beneath. By focusing only on the sequence of event, thought, and behaviour, we risk overlooking how that event was lived in the adolescent's body and relationships.

This is the difference between understanding what happened and understanding how it was felt. Both matter. But if we lose sight of the feeling, we lose our way.

I've seen many adolescents accept the idea that there might be a feeling underneath the thought, some spark that comes first. But, soon after, they often ask, 'So what could it be, then?' or 'What kind of feelings happen before that sort of thought?' These are hard questions to answer. Even if we could name the likely feeling, it wouldn't matter unless that feeling can actually be felt. Unless it lands in the body, in the psyche, in the self, no real shift in the OCD process is likely to happen. Intellectual insight alone is rarely enough. The change comes when the feeling becomes emotionally thinkable.

Here, the threads of the chapter draw together: whether we speak of Bion's preconceptions, Bollas's unthought known, Klein's projective identifications, or Freud's repressions, each points to the same truth – that the thought is rarely the beginning. To work with adolescents in the grip of intrusive images, we must look not just for the story of the thought but for the spark of the feeling that preceded it.

In the next chapter, we will turn our attention to the dominant psychological intervention models currently used for OCD in adolescence. While these models often begin with the thought, we now ask: how do they respond to the feeling beneath? What do they offer, and what might they miss, when the emotional weight of the symptom is not fully acknowledged?

References

Bion, W. R. (1962). *Learning from experience.* London: Heinemann.

Bion, W. R. (1970). *Attention and interpretation.* London: Tavistock.

Bollas, C. (1987). *The shadow of the object: Psychoanalysis of the unthought known.* London: Free Association Books.

Fonagy, P., Gergely, G., Jurist, E., & Target, M. (2002). *Affect regulation, mentalization and the development of the self.* London: Karnac.

Freud, S. (1915). Repression. In J. Strachey (Ed. & Trans.), *The standard edition of the complete psychological works of Sigmund Freud* (Vol. 14, pp. 141–158). London: Hogarth Press.

Klein, M. (1946). Notes on some schizoid mechanisms. *The International Journal of Psychoanalysis, 27,* 99–110.

LeDoux, J. E. (1996). *The emotional brain: The mysterious underpinnings of emotional life.* New York: Simon & Schuster.

Raichle, M. E. (2015). The brain's default mode network. *Annual Review of Neuroscience, 38,* 433–447. doi:10.1146/annurev-neuro-071013-014030.

Schore, A. N. (2003). *Affect dysregulation and disorders of the self.* New York: Norton.

Spillius, E., & O'Shaughnessy, E. (Eds.). (2012). *Projective identification: The fate of a concept.* London and New York: Routledge. doi:10.4324/9780203157220.

van der Kolk, B. (2014). *The body keeps the score: Brain, mind, and body in the healing of trauma.* New York: Viking.

Waska, R. (2021). *Projective identification: A contemporary introduction.* London and New York: Routledge. doi:10.4324/9781003112129.

Winnicott, D. W. (1974). Fear of breakdown. *International Review of Psycho-Analysis, 1,* 103–107.

Chapter 6

What We Know Works

As discussed throughout previous chapters, the treatment most often placed in front of young people with obsessive-compulsive disorder is cognitive behavioural therapy (CBT) and, at its heart, exposure response prevention (ERP). It is the psychological approach supported by the National Institute for Health and Care Excellence (NICE, 2005) in the UK, the American Psychiatric Association (APA, 2013), and the World Health Organization (WHO, 2019), among other international guidelines. Its effectiveness is supported by decades of careful research.

I have often seen the relief in families when ERP works well: when a ritual that once consumed hours collapses into minutes, and an adolescent realises they can begin to live again. The evidence is consistent. Young people who complete a structured course of ERP do better than those who rely on medication alone or on other therapies (Reid et al., 2021; Uhre et al., 2020; Tao et al., 2022). When it is delivered well, the effects can be striking and transformational. Intrusive thoughts lose their edge, rituals begin to loosen, and life starts to feel liveable again.

ERP has been studied across cultures, ages, and in young people with additional diagnoses. The principle is simple but mentally demanding: turn toward what is feared, resist the ritual, and stay with the anxiety that follows. For many adolescents, this can be transformative; not because the fear disappears, but because they discover it no longer has to dictate their lives.

How ERP Works

A thought arrives: intrusive, violent, shameful. It doesn't sit well with the adolescent. It may feel alien, outside their personality, even outside their sense of self. The mind treats it as dangerous. A surge of anxiety follows, a response to this perceived threat. To quieten the feeling, the adolescent turns to ritual, which can include and is not limited to, checking, confessing, washing, mentally neutralising. It works, briefly. The anxiety recedes, and a modicum of relief is felt. But the relief is short-lived. Worse, it reinforces the idea that the thought is dangerous and must be responded to with compulsion.

DOI: 10.4324/9781003729716-6

One of the most studied maintaining mechanisms is thought–action fusion: the belief that merely having a thought makes it more likely to happen, or is morally equivalent to acting on it (Shafran, Thordarson, & Rachman, 1996). Alongside this, inflated responsibility (Salkovskis, 1985), perfectionism, and intolerance of uncertainty have also been identified (OCCWG, 1997, 2005). From a CBT perspective, these are distortions to be tested. From a psycho-analytic perspective, as discussed in Chapter 3, they may be residues of early psychic life: omnipotence resurfacing, responsibility carried too soon, dread of mixed feelings. ERP alone may not explain these, but it creates the conditions in which they can be softened, symbolised, and worked through.

The way rituals take shape is rarely a matter of chance. Someone may find themselves praying ten times over, while another feels compelled to touch the table twenty times. On the surface, almost any act that blunts the anxiety could suffice. Yet, in practice, the form tends to echo the nature of the fear beneath. A prayer can feel like an appeal for moral safety, while endless washing carries the hope of scrubbing away shame. Counting rituals impose order on inner chaos. In adolescence, when puberty stirs sexuality, morality, and responsibility, rituals cluster around those very shifts. Magical thinking, so ordinary in childhood, returns with force, the belief that a thought might cause an event, or that only ritual can contain desire.

How ERP Changes Belief

ERP works not only by interrupting behaviour but also by reshaping belief through lived experience. It shows the adolescent that thoughts are not actions, that uncertainty can be tolerated, and that danger is not inevitable. Essentially, it helps the adolescent's mind learn: 'This thought is uncomfortable, but it means nothing. I can tolerate this discomfort.'

Instead of escaping the thought, the young person leans in. Through exposure, they face the feared image or situation; through response prevention, they resist the ritual. Anxiety rises sharply at first, which is often why engagement is hard. But, over time, the feared catastrophe does not arrive, the thought loses its sting, and a new belief takes root: 'I can bear this. I do not need the ritual.'

When I sit with adolescents during exposure, I often notice the exact moment their anxiety peaks. They glance at me to see if I believe they can survive it. That look is as important as the exercise itself. Bion (1962) emphasised the role of containment in tolerating emotional pain. ERP in practice often relies as much on this containing function as on the behavioural protocol.

From one angle, this is exposure therapy in distilled form. From another, it is re-education in meaning. By standing in the presence of what once had to be expelled or neutralised, the adolescent learns that fear itself is survivable. For those who can tolerate the process, the change can be profound.

ERP: Tool, Not Total Solution

ERP is a tool. It is structured, effective, and for many young people profoundly empowering. But harm is done when it is treated as sufficient in itself.

Intrusive thoughts are not only cognitive distortions that trigger compulsions. They are also emotional events which are charged with unconscious dynamics, relational ruptures, and symbolic fears (see Chapter 5). If we only target the thought, we risk missing the person who is thinking it.

ERP offers behaviour change. Deeper work offers psychic integration. Other approaches are beginning to widen the field. Acceptance and commitment therapy (ACT) encourages a more flexible stance toward thoughts through mindfulness and values. Inference-based therapy (IBT) examines the reasoning processes that generate obsessions. Mindfulness-based CBT (MBCBT) invites non-judgemental awareness of mental events. None yet rival ERP's empirical weight, but each reminds us the landscape is evolving and that no single method should be mistaken for the whole truth.

At the same time, it is important to remember why ERP remains the gold standard. Its effects have been consistently demonstrated across trials, across cultures, across developmental stages, and in diverse service contexts. It is the only approach with sufficient evidence to be considered first-line treatment worldwide.

The Symbolic Shape of Rituals

ERP shows, very concretely, that compulsions can be dismantled by lived experience. Yet the sheer persistence of some rituals only really makes sense when we think about their symbolic place in an adolescent's inner life. From a psychoanalytic point of view, compulsions are not random habits at all, but fragments of meaning. The shape a ritual takes can often point back toward the feeling it is trying to manage.

I remember reading Klein's *The Psycho-Analysis of Children* and coming across her case of Ruth, a 10-year-old who insisted on tucking in her dolls before being tightly tucked in herself (Klein, 1932). Klein saw this as Ruth's way of checking and managing her own aggression. At the time, it struck me as a bit of an imaginative leap. I suspect many non-analytic therapists would think the same. Yet, over the years, as I began to notice how anger, when it is not consciously owned, seems to intensify compulsions, it made more and more sense. When rituals are interrupted or done 'wrong', the secondary anger can flare with just as much force. Klein's interpretation, which once felt far-fetched, began to feel almost obvious.

More recent research quietly supports this. Barcaccia et al. (2022) found a significant association between trait anger and obsessive-compulsive symptoms, particularly in checking behaviours. Other studies have shown that self-reported anger correlates with OCD severity and that suppressing anger can maintain symptoms (Cludius et al., 2020; Ince & Kandil, 2018). All this suggests that unacknowledged anger fuels compulsions, a finding that feels deeply familiar in the clinic.

In therapy, I have noticed that intrusive thoughts and rituals often tighten when anger goes unexpressed. It is rarely clear at the start, but by the middle phase it becomes apparent. When adolescents begin to notice their own irritation – frustration with parents, teachers, even with me – and can name it without shame, the compulsions often start to loosen. A little more assertiveness, a bit of honest protest, and the ritual that once felt immovable begins to fade. This kind of practice-based evidence gives quiet credit to Klein's early intuition.

Meltzer (1967, 1992) widened Klein's idea. He suggested compulsions are not only about anger but about a whole range of unbearable feelings. Sometimes the adolescent is not aware of them; other times they know them but fear what might happen if they surface. I have seen rituals tighten not only around anger but around guilt, shame, rejection, and tenderness. Meltzer never listed these states explicitly, but in practice they are there, woven through the work. Compulsions can be ways of managing emotions that feel unsafe to have.

When adolescents and I map their OCD together, we often begin with 'stress'. But, as the work deepens, that word turns out to be a placeholder covering guilt, sadness, vulnerability, uselessness. This, I think, is very much in keeping with Meltzer's notion that compulsions defend against a range of disallowed feelings. Empirical work echoes this too. Shame and guilt correlate with OCD severity, particularly in symptom clusters that are self-evaluative (Laving et al., 2023; Hendriks, Haling, & Schoneveld, 2022). Difficulties with emotional regulation have been found to predict both symptom intensity and insight (Barcaccia et al., 2022; Yazici & Yazici, 2019). What this means clinically is that mapping OCD with a young person often becomes a map of their emotional life, not just the feelings that shout but the ones that hide. Rituals, in that light, can look like armour against emotion itself.

When I began reading more widely, I was struck by how little had been written about OCD in this symbolic way. The imbalance is stark: on one side, the vast empirical literature on CBT and ERP; on the other, the psychoanalytic view – sporadic, almost apologetic. Perhaps it should not have surprised me, but it did. The dynamics are visible in any clinic on a Tuesday morning, yet the literature scarcely names them. Reviews confirm this imbalance: CBT dominates the evidence base, while psychoanalytic contributions remain mostly conceptual (Steele et al., 2025; Cassin & Rector, 2012).

Gregory Rizzolo is one of the few recent writers to reopen the conversation. He places compulsions in the realm of volition, the capacity to choose and act, and shows how rituals manage anxieties about autonomy and identification (Rizzolo, 2019, 2023). His work gave me language for something I had sensed but not named. Others, like Parish (2022), have explored the cultural and symbolic meanings of ritual. These ideas may sound abstract at first, especially if one's training has been steeped in CBT, but over time they ring true to what we see daily in clinic.

As I have written earlier, adolescence is already a conflict between separation and dependency. Sometimes OCD feels like a detour around that struggle. One boy told me he could not date because no partner would ever understand. Another said he hated asking his parents to accommodate him but could not stop. On the surface, these are practical statements. Underneath, they hint at fear of intimacy, of responsibility, of growing up. Rizzolo's work gave me permission to lean into those conversations, to shift the focus from the ritual itself to the adolescent task beneath it.

Around that time I discovered Darian Leader. I did not always follow every argument, but I was drawn to his way of thinking – less diagnostic, more curious about meaning. His book *Hands: What We Do with Them – and Why* (2016) was not about OCD, yet it spoke directly to it. Leader warns that if we treat OCD purely as behaviour to be modified, we risk flattening the very conflicts that give it life. ERP, by design, targets the surface ritual, not the emotional world that created it. For Leader, rituals are messages, signs of conflicts that have not yet found another way to speak.

This is something I feel again and again in practice. Young people can list every step of their ritual, but when I ask what feeling comes with it, the room falls quiet. The act is easier to describe than the emotion it suppresses. One girl told me her nightly checking was 'just something I have to do'. Only later did frustration and disappointment with her family begin to show. The ritual seemed to be doing double duty, warding off intrusive fears while holding down feelings too risky to express. That is when I began to think in terms of the psychic retreat: the ritual as a substitute for a conversation that cannot yet happen.

Fonagy's work adds another layer. If Leader warns against treating rituals as surface, Fonagy shows what can happen when the feelings inside them are finally spoken. In his case of Glen, a 15-year-old consumed by ritual, analysis made possible a space for emotion that had been trapped inside the compulsion (Fonagy, 1999). Once symbolised, those feelings could be thought about rather than enacted. I have seen this too; young people who at first seem to be 'nothing but ritual', their days packed with checking or counting. But when a feeling breaks through, grief, guilt, shame, the ritual's purpose suddenly makes sense. It had been both prison and protection.

Gabbard (2001) described compulsions as a form of undoing. CBT says they lower anxiety; Gabbard agrees, but adds that they also cancel out angry or guilty impulses before they fully take shape. A boy who apologises compulsively may be trying to undo an imagined aggression; a girl who rewrites homework may be scrubbing out anger toward her teacher. These gestures are not just about anxiety reduction, they are attempts to erase inner experience.

King (2017) wrote a psychodynamic chapter in a book that focused on the phenomenology of OCD. In it, he reflected on how OCD has been understood from a psychodynamic perspective, exploring how these experiences can often trace back to childhood. While some of the older terminology –

like 'anal-sadistic' or 'Oedipal' – feels dated now, the underlying idea still resonates: that adolescent compulsions can revisit early struggles around autonomy, control, rivalry, and guilt. I see echoes of this often. Rituals around order and contamination can replay early conflicts over control and mess; checking and confession can rehearse old tensions to do with loyalty and blame. The ritual, then, may be less about the catastrophe imagined in the present, and more about an attempt to repair something in the past.

Leib (2001) offered a case combining CBT, medication, and analysis. What stood out was not the integration itself but her insistence that compulsions carry meaning. CBT and medication reduced symptoms, but analytic work explained why those rituals had taken hold in the first place. I have seen this too: medication and ERP can steady the ground, but unless we leave space for meaning, something essential is missed. One adolescent I worked with improved with ERP and an SSRI (selective serotonin reuptake inhibitor), but therapy only deepened when he realised that checking felt like punishment, a way to manage guilt he could not articulate.

Kempke and Luyten (2007) built a bridge between the two worlds. They described compulsions as symbolic attempts at affect regulation. Rituals, in their view, do not simply reduce anxiety but manage overwhelming feeling. One boy once told me his counting helped 'calm the storm inside'. His phrase, not mine. It struck me as a perfect meeting point between analytic and CBT frames. For him, the ritual was both behaviour and symbol.

Taken together, these writers show that compulsions are never random. Whether we see them as symbolic acts, defences against unbearable emotion, diversions from autonomy, messages of unspoken conflict, containers for feeling, undoing gestures, or replays of early struggles, the point is the same: rituals are saturated with meaning.

And, in practice, recognising that symbolic layer does not conflict with ERP, it deepens it. It helps explain why some adolescents engage readily, while others resist or relapse. The ritual, once seen as empty repetition, begins to speak.

When ERP Does Not Help

Initial Barriers

ERP does not always work. Many adolescents are unable to complete a full course, and the reasons are varied. Sometimes the difficulty lies on the surface: the task feels too frightening, or the young person cannot yet take the positive risk of tolerating anxiety without ritual. At first, it is tempting to frame this as lack of motivation. In practice, the obstacles are more complex. In a recent narrative review by Mukai et al. (2025), which included reviewing 24 studies, the authors found that dropout is rarely about simple unwillingness or lack of motivation; it often reflects an amalgamation of developmental, cognitive, and contextual factors that shape how exposure is experienced. For some, limitations in cognitive flexibility or intolerance of uncertainty make ERP feel overwhelming and too distressing. For others, family dynamics interfere with engagement. These nuances remind us that non-completion is not failure, but a signal to adapt our approach.

Before concluding that ERP has failed, the clinician must consider a series of questions. Has the rationale been explained in language the adolescent can truly digest, and pitched at their developmental rather than chronological age? Have the parents been brought on board, and are they able to support the exposures at home without becoming too distressed themselves? Has enough containment been offered before asking the adolescent to step directly into fear? At times, the difficulty is not with ERP itself but with the way it is introduced, explained, or supported.

I'd add, too, that what the young person is struggling with is not always fear but shame. Intrusive thoughts with a violent or taboo edge can be almost impossible to speak aloud, even in a clinical room. Silence here is often shaped by culture and upbringing. I've met families where 'people who think such things' are openly condemned, which leaves the adolescent afraid of being judged not only as anxious but as dangerous, even contaminated. And while we may work hard to normalise such thoughts, the internal shame can still feel unbearable. At those times, it isn't simply the exposure that cannot be tolerated, it is the act of giving the thought voice, letting it exist between oneself and another.

Secondary Gains and Hesitation

The idea that symptoms can carry unconscious benefits has long been recognised across traditions in Freud's writing, in later psychodynamic theory, in psychosomatic medicine, and even among behavioural clinicians who note the reinforcing power of illness roles. In the context of OCD, ERP sometimes collides with this dynamic. Freud (1926) spoke of 'secondary gain', and later psychoanalysts such as Steiner (1993) elaborated how retreat into symptom can preserve a fragile sense of self.

For some adolescents, remaining in the position of being unwell carries hidden advantages: exemption from expectation, a ready explanation for difficulties, or an identity that draws care. OCD can even take on a paradoxical value, a fragile sense of specialness distinct from peers.

For these young people, the compulsion is not only feared but also clung to. The rituals may offer not just protection against anxiety but a structure that makes life manageable. While it is always hard for an adolescent to imagine a world without OCD, sometimes the prospect is more frightening than the disorder itself. At one level, this is because of the sheer intensity of anxiety that exposures provoke. But, at another, it is because OCD has become woven into the fabric of identity. It explains quirks and limitations, but also achievements and survival. It provides a narrative, 'this is why I am the way I am', and in that sense it functions as a stabiliser of self.

Taking that away can feel less like relief than like a threat of disintegration. To relinquish OCD may mean relinquishing the very story that holds their world together. Even if this is not consciously acknowledged, it can explain why some adolescents resist ERP or abandon it after initial attempts. For them, OCD is not just a problem to be solved; it is a scaffolding of identity. From that perspective, it makes sense why someone might prefer to keep the rituals rather than risk the psychic collapse of losing them.

I am reminded of working with a 15-year-old boy who had lived with OCD since primary school. His rituals centred on checking locks, power sockets, and switches. When we first spoke about ERP, he nodded politely and seemed to understand the rationale. Yet, as we progressed, his anxiety surged. After one session, where he successfully resisted a compulsion, he returned looking unsettled. 'It felt weird,' he admitted. 'Like ... if I don't do it, then who am I? I've been like this forever. It's just me.'

For him, the ritual was not only a shield against anxiety but a marker of identity. It explained why he stayed up late, why he was exhausted at school, even why he sometimes felt different from friends. The thought of losing it left him exposed, as if without OCD there would be no story to make sense of his struggles. ERP had not failed him at the level of technique, it had touched something deeper: the fear that dismantling rituals meant dismantling the fragile scaffolding that gave him coherence.

Yet even when psychoeducation is clear, parents are supportive, and motivation is high, ERP can still falter. This is where the literature remains thin. The deeper question is not only whether ERP is pitched at the right level, but what kind of internal relationship the adolescent has with their OCD.

It is this relationship – their psychic stance toward the obsession and the ritual – that determines whether ERP can be used as a tool or whether it rebounds as another source of persecution. As argued in earlier chapters, rituals do not exist in isolation. They are part of a lived relationship the adolescent has with their own mind. Some may hate their OCD yet also feel it provides a strange comfort, even a private identity. Others may experience rituals as non-negotiable facts, less a choice than a place they live inside.

These are not superficial quirks. They are psychic positions: organising stances that shape how OCD is experienced and how treatment is received.

Evidence of Dropout and Relapse

A meta-analysis by Ong et al. (2016) reported a weighted mean dropout rate of 14.7 per cent. When refusal to begin treatment was included, attrition rose to 18.7 per cent. Although these figures are comparable to those of other treatments, the authors noted that clinician anxieties about ERP being too distressing may still limit its use in practice. I find this to be a fine line to tread. On the one hand, as clinicians, we cannot collude with fear; I know from experience how easy it is to become caught up in the anxiety of OCD and risk practising in ways that are inadvertently anti-therapeutic. We have to model confidence, hope, and optimism that ERP can work. On the other hand, we must be mindful of where the adolescent is in relation to their OCD. If this is their whole world, if they have become immersed in it as a means of functioning in a locked down and claustrophobic state (what I later describe as the claustrum position), then forcing ERP too soon can be not only distressing but at times unethical.

Long-term follow-up studies also paint a sobering picture. In one seven-to-nine-year follow-up, nearly 40 per cent of young people treated with CBT, including ERP, still met full criteria for OCD, and almost 70 per cent had developed another psychiatric disorder (Fatori et al., 2020). Early intervention, while vital, did not reliably predict lasting recovery. Of course, a lot can change in seven to nine years. Unimaginable adverse experiences and relational disruptions can occur, so it is important to remember that ERP was never going to be the panacea for all adolescent OCD. That said, given the high proportion who continued to meet diagnostic criteria, we have to be curious about what specifically was happening for this 40 per cent. Once again, I find myself drawn to the psychic relationship they had with their OCD.

Qualitative research adds further insight to these numbers. Interviews with adolescents who had a formal diagnosis of OCD suggest that some disengaged not because they lacked insight, but because the process felt alien, emotionally unanchored, or misaligned with how their distress was experienced (Krebs, Heyman, & Mataix-Cols, 2024). Others describe feeling unheard, or that therapy failed to adapt to the nuances of their OCD. These voices remind us that therapeutic success is not just about compliance or symptom reduction, but about whether the work feels meaningful, safe, and connected to the adolescent's lived reality.

In my own practice, I have seen how the very same protocol that frees one adolescent can feel unreachable to another, not because ERP is faulty, but because their stance toward thought and ritual is different. This is not simply a matter of compliance or technique. It points to the emotional and developmental challenges adolescents face when asked to confront their most shame-driven and distressing thoughts. These figures underscore the need for approaches that are more nuanced, flexible, and symbolically attuned, frameworks that take seriously not just the symptom but the psychic position from which the adolescent meets it.

Closing Bridge

ERP teaches us that fear can be endured, that rituals can be resisted, and that the mind can relearn safety. Yet there remain adolescents for whom even this is not enough, those whose intrusive thoughts are experienced less as distortions than as states of being, sealed off from contact. For ERP to reach its full effectiveness, we sometimes need to first navigate the psychic architecture of their difficulties.

In my own practice, I have often found that what makes or breaks ERP is not the protocol itself, but the position from which the adolescent meets it. Some can use ERP directly, discovering that fear can be survived. Others encounter ERP as persecutory, irrelevant, or simply unworkable, because their relationship to the thought and to themselves is organised at a deeper level.

The chapters that follow set out to describe these stances; what I call psychic positions. They are not new diagnoses, nor replacements for ERP, but clinical textures that help us understand why the same technique liberates one adolescent and falters with another. By beginning with the claustrum, we enter the first of these positions, where withdrawal into ritual provides psychic survival but at the cost of growth and contact. From there, each position opens a way of listening beneath the surface of symptoms and of pacing ERP so it can be used to greatest effect, without unnecessary distress, while deepening our grasp of the relationship a young person has with their OCD. ERP therefore remains essential, but it gains its true force when situated within an understanding of psychic position. It is this movement – from evidence-based technique to the symbolic stance of the adolescent – that forms the threshold we now cross in Chapter 7.

References

American Psychiatric Association (APA). (2013). *Diagnostic and statistical manual of mental disorders* (5th ed.). Arlington, VA: American Psychiatric Publishing. doi:10.1176/appi.books.9780890425596.

Barcaccia, B., Cervin, M., Pallini, S., Couyoumdjian, A., Mancini, F., & Pozza, A. (2022). Whom are you mad at? Anger and revenge in obsessive–compulsive symptoms during adolescence. *Journal of Obsessive–Compulsive and Related Disorders*, 35, 100763. doi:10.1016/j.jocrd.2022.100763.

Bion, W. R. (1962). *Learning from experience*. London: Heinemann.

Cassin, S. E., & Rector, N. A. (2012). Psychological models of obsessive compulsive and spectrum disorders. In G. Steketee (Ed.), *Oxford handbook of obsessive compulsive and spectrum disorders* (chap. 41). Oxford: Oxford University Press. doi:10.1093/oxfordhb/9780195376210.013.0041.

Cludius, B., Mannsfeld, A. K., Schmidt, A. F., & Jelinek, L. (2020). Anger and aggressiveness in obsessive–compulsive disorder (OCD) and the mediating role of responsibility, non-acceptance of emotions, and social desirability. *European Archives of Psychiatry and Clinical Neuroscience*, 271(6), 1179–1191. doi:10.1007/s00406-020-01199-8.

Fatori, D., Polanczyk, G. V., de Morais, R. M. C. B., & Asbahr, F. R. (2020). Long-term outcome of children and adolescents with obsessive–compulsive disorder: A 7–9-year follow-up of a randomized clinical trial. *European Child & Adolescent Psychiatry*, 29, 1613–1616. doi:10.1007/s00787-019-01457-8.

Fonagy, P. (1999). The transgenerational transmission of holocaust trauma: Lessons learned from the analysis of an adolescent with obsessive–compulsive disorder. *Attachment & Human Development*, 1(1), 92–114. doi:10.1080/14616739900134041.

Freud, S. (1926). *Inhibitions, symptoms and anxiety* (J. Strachey, Trans.). London: Hogarth Press.

Gabbard, G. O. (2001). Psychoanalytically informed approaches to the treatment of obsessive–compulsive disorder. *Psychoanalytic Inquiry*, 21(2), 208–221. doi:10.1080/07351692109348932.

Hendriks, J., Haling, M. S., & Schoneveld, K. (2022). Childhood disorder: Dysregulated self-conscious emotions? Psychopathological correlates of implicit and explicit shame and guilt in clinical and non-clinical children and adolescents. *Frontiers in Psychology*, 13, 822725. doi:10.3389/fpsyg.2022.822725.

Ince, C., & Kandil, S. (2018). Anger level and depression relation in children and adolescents with obsessive–compulsive disorder. *Anatolian Journal of Psychiatry*, 19(3), 307–313. doi:10.5455/apd.279638.

Kempke, S., & Luyten, P. (2007). Psychodynamic and cognitive–behavioral approaches of obsessive–compulsive disorder: Is it time to work through our ambivalence? *Bulletin of the Menninger Clinic*, 71(4), 291–311. doi:10.1521/bumc.2007.71.4.291.

King, R. A. (2017). Psychodynamic perspectives on OCD. In C. Pittenger (Ed.), *Obsessive-compulsive disorder: Phenomenology, pathophysiology, and treatment* (pp. 65–72). Oxford: Oxford University Press. doi:10.1093/med/9780190228163.003.0007.

Klein, M. (1932). *The psycho-analysis of children*. London: Hogarth Press.

Krebs, G., Heyman, I., & Mataix-Cols, D. (2024). Navigating recovery in childhood OCD: A qualitative analysis of barriers and facilitators. *Child and Adolescent Psychiatry and Mental Health*, 18, article 160. doi:10.1186/s13034-024-00851-8.

Laving, M., Foroni, F., Ferrari, M., Turner, C., & Yap, K. (2023). The association between OCD and shame: A systematic review and meta-analysis. *British Journal of Clinical Psychology*, 62, 28–52. doi:10.1111/bjc.12392.

Leader, D. (2016). *Hands: What we do with them – and why.* London: Hamish Hamilton.

Leib, P. (2001). A psychoanalytic view of obsessive–compulsive disorder: A case study. *Journal of Psychotherapy Integration*, 11(3), 417–432.

Meltzer, D. (1967). *The psycho-analytical process.* London: Heinemann.

Meltzer, D. (1992). *The claustrum: An investigation of claustrophobic phenomena.* London: Karnac Books.

Mukai, K., Kyosuke, Y., Ogino, S., Hosoi, Y., Hayashida, K., & Matsunaga, H. (2025). Benefits and barriers associated with using cognitive–behavioral therapy to treat obsessive–compulsive disorder: A narrative review. *Frontiers in Psychiatry*, 16, 1593384. doi:10.3389/fpsyt.2025.1593384.

National Institute for Health and Care Excellence (NICE). (2005; updated 2024). *Obsessive-compulsive disorder and body dysmorphic disorder: Treatment (Clinical guideline 31).* London: NICE.

Obsessive Compulsive Cognitions Working Group (OCCWG). (1997). Cognitive assessment of obsessive-compulsive disorder. *Behaviour Research and Therapy*, 35(7), 667–681. doi:10.1016/S0005-7967(97)00017-X

Obsessive Compulsive Cognitions Working Group (OCCWG). (2005). Psychometric validation of the obsessive belief questionnaire and interpretation of intrusions inventory—Part 2: Factor analyses and testing of a brief version. *Behaviour Research and Therapy*, 43(11), 1527–1542. doi:10.1016/j.brat.2004.07.010.

Ong, C. W., Clyde, J. L., Bluett, E. J., Levin, M. E., & Twohig, M. P. (2016). Dropout rates in exposure with response prevention for obsessive–compulsive disorder: What do the data really say? *Journal of Anxiety Disorders*, 40, 29–36. doi:10.1016/j.janxdis.2016.04.001.

Parish, J. (2022). The spectral material culture in ordinary life: Re-imagining obsessive-compulsive disorder (OCD). *The Sociological Review*, 70(1), 117–132. doi:10.1177/00380261211049034.

Reid, J. E., Laws, K. R., Drummond, L., Vismara, M., Grancini, B., Mpavaenda, D., & Fineberg, N. A. (2021). Cognitive behavioural therapy with exposure and response prevention in the treatment of obsessive–compulsive disorder: A systematic review and meta-analysis of randomised controlled trials. *Comprehensive Psychiatry*, 106, 152223. doi:10.1016/j.comppsych.2021.152223.

Rizzolo, G. S. (2019). The life cycle (without regression). *The Psychoanalytic Study of the Child*, 72, 207–227. doi:10.1080/00797308.2019.1558624.

Rizzolo, G. S. (2023). Obsessions and compulsions: A lifespan perspective. *Journal of the American Psychoanalytic Association*, 71(3), 445–487. doi:10.1177/00030651231 182441.

Salkovskis, P. M. (1985). Obsessional–compulsive problems: A cognitive–behavioural analysis. *Behaviour Research and Therapy*, 23(5), 571–583. doi:10.1016/0005-7967 (85)90105–90106.

Sarawgi, S., & Mathews, R. E. (2025). Emotion regulation in pediatric obsessive–compulsive disorder and related interventions: A scoping review. *Children*, 12(4), 400. doi:10.3390/children12040400.

Shafran, R., Thordarson, D. S., & Rachman, S. (1996). Thought–action fusion in obsessive–compulsive disorder. *Journal of Anxiety Disorders*, 10(5), 379–391. doi:10.1016/0887-6185(96)00018–00017.

Steele, D. W., Kanaan, G., Caputo, E. L., Freeman, J. B., Brannan, E. H., Balk, E. M., Trikalinos, T. A., & Adam, G. P. (2025). Treatment of obsessive–compulsive disorder in children and youth: A meta-analysis. *Pediatrics*, 155(3). doi:10.1542/peds.2024-068992.

Steiner, J. (1993). *Psychic retreats: Pathological organizations in psychotic, neurotic and borderline patients*. London and New York: Routledge.

Tao, Y., Li, H., Li, L., Zhang, H., Xu, H., Zhang, H., Zou, S., Deng, F., Huang, L., Wang, Y., & Wang, X. (2022). Comparing the efficacy of pharmacological and psychological treatment, alone and in combination, in children and adolescents with obsessive–compulsive disorder: A network meta-analysis. *Journal of Psychiatric Research*, 148, 95–102. doi:10.1016/j.jpsychires.2022.01.057.

Uhre, C. F., Uhre, V. F., Lønfeldt, N., Pretzmann, L., Vangkilde, S., Plessen, K. J., Gluud, C., Jakobsen, J. C., & Pagsberg, A. K. (2020). Systematic review and meta-analysis: Cognitive-behavioural therapy for obsessive–compulsive disorder in children and adolescents. *Journal of the American Academy of Child & Adolescent Psychiatry*, 59(1), 64–77. doi:10.1016/j.jaac.2019.08.480.

World Health Organization (WHO). (2019). *The WHO special initiative for mental health (2019–2023): Universal health coverage for mental health*. Geneva: WHO.

Yazici, K. U., & Yazici, I. P. (2019). Decreased theory of mind skills, increased emotion dysregulation and insight levels in adolescents diagnosed with obsessive–compulsive disorder. *Nordic Journal of Psychiatry*, 73(7), 462–469. doi:10.1080/08039488.2019.1652341.

Chapter 7

The Threshold

Up to this point, this book has traced intrusive thoughts in adolescence from several directions. We began with their raw impact in the consulting room and on the immediate family, noticing how reassurance can soothe only momentarily and often perpetuates the cycle of obsessive-compulsive disorder (OCD). We then looked at how OCD is typically defined by diagnostic manuals, and why those categorical maps so often miss the lived reality of young people.

From there, I introduced the idea that residues of infancy resurface under the pressures of puberty – omnipotence of thought, magical control, the early burden of responsibility – and showed how these mechanisms reappear as intrusive fears and compulsive rituals. We explored the emotional undercurrents of intrusive thoughts, where unprocessed feelings find expression in symbols too painful to own directly. And, most recently, I reviewed what contemporary services can reliably offer: cognitive behavioural therapy (CBT) with exposure and response prevention (ERP), an approach supported by decades of outcome data.

Taken together, these chapters present a dual picture: the strength of structured interventions, their clarity and proven benefit; and the stubborn fact that not every adolescent can use them, that symptoms often carry symbolic weight beyond the reach of protocol. It is here, at this meeting point between technique and meaning, that we arrive at the threshold.

Adolescence itself is a threshold: between childhood and adulthood, dependence and autonomy, bodily change and psychic reorganisation. It is also a threshold in the consulting room, where families arrive expecting certainty yet leave with questions, and where clinicians often feel suspended between guidance and humility. For me, therapy at this point is not about rushing through the doorway but about pausing long enough to notice what the threshold reveals.

Compulsions and Symbolic Life

Obsessions and compulsions deserve equal attention. They are not simply habits to be extinguished but symbolic gestures in their own right. A boy

DOI: 10.4324/9781003729716-7

who washes until his hands bleed may be scrubbing away shame or guilt as much as germs. A girl who repeats a prayer is not only neutralising a thought but attempting to repair an inner rupture she cannot yet name.

Magical thinking, often dismissed as childish, can be an adolescent's attempt to wrestle with morality and desire in a world complicated by technology and unspoken social rules. To treat compulsions only as behavioural loops is to miss their communicative force. At the threshold of psychoanalytic listening, rituals become a language: a way of expressing what words cannot carry.

The aim is not to unmask what these compulsions 'really mean', but to allow them to be seen as more than anxiety-reduction strategies. In this view, rituals are both symptoms and symbols; survival tools that also tell a story. When listened to in this way, they open the door to the deeper positions that follow.

When ERP Reaches Its Limits

Not every young person responds to exposure and response prevention (ERP), however well delivered. Some manage the exposures but relapse when treatment ends. Others cannot tolerate the exercises in the first place. Still others complete a course of therapy with apparent success, only to return months later, describing the same fears in a slightly altered form. For them, OCD is not a visitor to be evicted by technique alone; it is woven into their psychic fabric.

Relapse is not unusual in the follow-up studies, particularly when compulsions carry guilt, shame, or a symbolic burden (Fatori et al., 2020). I think of a young man who worked hard at contamination exposures and appeared to master them, only for the rituals to surge again when his grandfather died. What returned was not failure of technique but the underlying grief and anger that had always been present beneath the surface.

I have also seen adolescents declare themselves 'fine' after treatment, partly to meet parental or school expectations, yet still carry a private burden they cannot find words for. At those times, I have been left with a sinking feeling that we had missed the mark. The relapse is not evidence of resistance but a clue: the symptom is carrying something that behaviour alone cannot resolve.

To cross this threshold is therefore to move from symptom management into symbolic understanding. The question becomes not only "What technique works?" but also "What does this ritual mean? What position is the young person inhabiting as they live with their OCD?"

Foundations of Therapeutic Work

Before we begin identifying and working with different psychic positions in OCD, we must first think about the foundations of good therapeutic work.

Every clinician comes with their own orientation, and it is right that they do. Some are steeped in CBT, others in systemic or analytic traditions. Each brings its own strengths, and none owns the truth. What matters more than allegiance to a model is an awareness that effective practice rests on several shared therapeutic positions, attitudes of mind that sustain any treatment, whatever its form.

No framework – behavioural, systemic, or psychoanalytic – can stand without the living relationship between therapist and adolescent. However sophisticated our formulations become, change begins in the shared experience of two people sitting in a room, encountering what emerges between them. For me, this is where the real work starts, in the here and now, in how the young person uses the space, how they locate me in their inner world, and how I in turn find myself responding. These small, moment-to-moment exchanges are not incidental; they are the clinical terrain from which meaning grows. What unfolds between us often tells me more than the symptom history, how trust forms, how distance is maintained, where anxiety sits, and how it moves through the room.

Transference and countertransference sit at the centre of this work, not as abstract ideas, but as living evidence of the young person's psychic position. The feelings a young person evokes – helplessness, irritation, tenderness, confusion – are often the first clues to where they are internally. To notice these states without rushing to manage or interpret them is part of the discipline of the work. It demands patience and containment, qualities easily eroded in systems ruled by outcome measures and symptom graphs.

Tolerating uncertainty, working through rupture and repair, linking experiences, and staying close to the here and now form the quiet scaffolding of all good therapy. They allow us to think symbolically, to listen not only to what is said but to the emotional movement behind it. These are not techniques to apply. They are positions to hold.

It is important to acknowledge that this is not a practical or prescriptive way of working. Rather, it is a way of being in the room and organising the experiences that unfold in front of us. This approach should not become the only way to work with someone, but I do believe it is essential to hold on to these assets in order to make sense of what is happening, especially when it comes to understanding the psychic position a young person may be occupying.

Tolerating Uncertainty

Adolescent OCD often pulls both therapist and family toward the false safety of certainty: a diagnosis, a protocol, a reassurance. Yet the work depends on staying with what is not yet known. This is not passivity, but disciplined waiting, the capacity to think while not knowing, to resist explanation until something living takes shape. When we rush to define, we often foreclose the very meanings we hope to uncover.

This is one of the more challenging aspects to hold, particularly within systems that offer limited sessions and demand specific goals. We are expected to justify our work with measurable outcomes and daily data. But immediate interpretation can be a form of dismissal. I have learned that if I jump too quickly into explanation or normalisation, especially with adolescents presenting with familiar intrusive thoughts, contamination fears, or inappropriate sexual content, I risk missing something vital. These presentations may be my seventh or eighth of the month, but each young person deserves the space to let their experience unfold organically.

Even when something feels familiar, allowing it time to grow within the session helps a clearer picture emerge. More importantly, it prevents us from projecting our own understanding onto the young person's experience before they have had a chance to think about it themselves. This reminds me of Wilfred Bion's emphasis in *Learning from Experience* on helping the patient to think for themselves, rather than thinking on their behalf. Bion writes that the therapist must tolerate frustration and resist the impulse to provide ready-made thoughts, allowing the patient to develop their own capacity to think (Bion, 1962).

This is difficult enough in one-to-one work, but it becomes even more challenging when working with children and adolescents who are embedded within family systems. In these cases, the therapist is not only holding uncertainty for the young person in front of them, but also modelling that tolerance to the family, who may understandably be seeking quick fixes and clear answers. Saying 'we have to wait and see' is rarely satisfying, and is often met with anxiety or frustration. Yet it is essential to highlight the importance of not rushing in, not making assumptions, and not holding rigid preconceptions about what is happening. This is not just in the best interest of the young person, but is also a necessary stance for the therapist to take.

It is imperative to recognise that this is a demanding task. The ability to model confidence in not knowing, and to tolerate uncertainty, is not a passive stance. It is an active therapeutic position, and one that can help others begin to do the same.

Transference and Countertransference

Every therapeutic session carries projection. The young person places us somewhere inside their inner world. Sometimes, we are experienced as safe and kind. Sometimes, as cold, judging, or even dangerous. I might believe I am being the same person from session to session, yet adolescent one sees me as the best clinician ever, adolescent two sees me as persecutory, and adolescent three sees me as kind until the moment I gently challenge her. From my side, I haven't changed. I can't possibly be all these versions. What shifts are the projections being placed on me, and those are what the young person is reacting to.

These projections usually happen without words. Our own feelings in response become part of the clinical information: the irritation that comes after the tenth reassurance, the sense of being tested, the sudden warmth or exhaustion that seems to come from nowhere. All of these can be communications from the unconscious.

For clinicians who work mostly in cognitive or behavioural frameworks, this way of paying attention can sound vague or soft. But these processes exist whether or not we look at them. They run beneath the surface of every session. We only gain some choice about them when we become curious and bring them into awareness.

To use our countertransference well means thinking about the feelings that get stirred in us and asking what they might be showing about the young person's inner world. It doesn't mean acting on them or pushing them away. It's a constant, moving process that changes from moment to moment as therapy unfolds.

The skill, I think, is keeping a sort of meta-awareness of the self. Am I feeling this because the young person has touched something personal in me, or because something alive is happening between us right now? Once I have a sense of that, I can ask the next question: would it help to share this with them at this point in time? What am I hoping might come from it?

Sometimes, I notice myself feeling distant or cut off. Have I lost interest, or are they pulling away? When it feels right, I might say quietly, 'I notice I'm feeling a bit distant from you. Do you feel that too, or is that just me?' Other times, it's frustration that appears. I remember one young person who answered every question with a calm 'I don't know.' After a while, I said that I was starting to feel frustrated and wondered if that might be how they felt when trying to understand their OCD. The session changed instantly. It became more alive. We could both feel something real happening in the room.

When we start to look at the textures of the room and think about which psychic position someone might be in, our own emotional responses become essential. Being tuned in to the countertransference and to the transferential pattern that is unfolding is the compass for this work. If we want to make evidence-based interpretations about position, we have to use ourselves as the instrument. Our feelings, our shifts in attention, the moments we lose interest or feel pulled too close, all offer small but vital clues about where the young person is standing internally.

Rupture and Repair

Therapeutic ruptures when working with adolescents are inevitable. What matters most is our ability to repair them. Sometimes, it is obvious that a young person is upset by what we have said or by something we haven't said at all. Other times, it is much harder to see. Many adolescents will hide their anger or hurt. They take enormous risks when they show us emotion of any kind, whether it is frustration, longing, curiosity, anger, or sadness.

Mistakes will happen. They are part of the work. When a young person with OCD is in the claustrum position there is often a pull in me to speed the session up, to make something happen. I might say something they are not ready to hear, and in doing so push them further into retreat. At other times, when I sense they are in a psychic retreat, I might comment on how they seem to withdraw into their compulsions when they feel rejected. Even though the observation is accurate, it may come too soon and they may not be able to bear it.

What matters is the repair. The ability to recognise the rupture, to take ownership of our part in it, and to acknowledge our limits. This is the foundation of all therapeutic work. Ruptures and repairs can happen continuously. They may unfold over several sessions or within the same hour. They are not always dramatic outbursts of anger or tears. Often, they are small, subtle moments that we barely notice.

Our task is to stay alert to these moments and to hold responsibility for them. That is what allows us to find our way back to the young person's psychic position, to understand what has happened in the space between us, and to keep the work alive.

Linking Experiences

Symptoms do not exist in isolation. They are part of a story the young person cannot yet tell. Linking experiences between past and present, thought and feeling, behaviour and meaning helps them begin to see their OCD as something that can be thought about rather than obeyed. A gentle question, offered at the right moment, can bring fragments together that have long remained separate.

This way of working is familiar to anyone trained in cognitive behavioural therapy, where we encourage young people to link their thoughts with their feelings, their bodily sensations, and their actions. The aim is to help them see that their experiences can be understood, and that they make emotional sense.

When we start to think about psychic positions, this linking becomes even more important. As sessions unfold, we can begin to notice the patterns that repeat, the way a particular feeling or event seems to set the OCD machinery turning. For example, a young person who retreats into compulsions whenever they feel criticised may be using a psychic retreat to manage the pain of shame. Making that link, at the right time, helps them begin to see what their mind is trying to do, rather than simply feeling trapped inside it.

Connecting experiences is like helping to create a story that makes sense of what has felt fragmented. It is the basis of meaning-making. Without these connections, we are left with pieces of a story that do not add up. What matters is that the links arise naturally. We cannot force them or impose meaning that isn't there. But when a genuine connection does appear, we need to notice it, to speak to it, and to reflect on it together.

In doing so, we not only deepen the young person's understanding of their OCD but also gain insight into the psychic position they are operating from. The pattern of links – what gets connected, what gets avoided, and when – tells us a great deal about where they are standing internally, and how we can best meet them there.

Here-and-Now Observation

Even in structured therapy, the present moment is the truest map of the mind. How the young person uses the session, how they sit, when they look away, what happens in silence, all reveal their position more clearly than any history. Describing these moments aloud can make the emotional field thinkable. A small comment such as, 'It feels a bit hard to think today, doesn't it?' can help turn atmosphere into understanding.

It is easy to become preoccupied with the past. While it matters to think about previous experiences, what is more therapeutically useful is to notice what is happening right now. Has a feeling appeared in the room? Has a memory suddenly come to mind? Focusing on what is unfolding in the present gives us a more living picture of what is moving inside them. The mind is never static. It is constantly shifting and re-forming. To follow it, we have to stay mobile too.

Being present in this way means commenting on what is happening in the room, on the tone, the atmosphere, and our own countertransference. These small observations are central to good therapy. They keep the work alive.

When it comes to understanding psychic positions, it is not enough to list how someone has responded to compulsions in the past. That can be useful background, but it does not tell us how they are positioned with us now. The real task is to capture the living quality of the relationship in front of us. A psychic position is not a historical record, it is a living stance. To see it clearly, we have to be in it with them, moment by moment, here and now.

Working with Positions

What follows in the next chapters is not a manual of techniques. The positions are not fixed or prescriptive, nor can they be spotted in a checklist at the first meeting. They are clinical textures, recognisable in the atmosphere of the room, in how the adolescent presents, and in what is evoked in the clinician.

This is where positions diverge most sharply from diagnostic categories. The DSM and ICD tell us what obsessions and compulsions look like. Positions tell us how they are lived. A classification may state 'contamination obsessions with washing rituals'. A position asks whether the washing is an act of penance, a retreat from feeling, or a safety device against imminent catastrophe. The behaviours may look identical; the psychic stance is not.

In my experience, every young person with obsessive-compulsive symptoms carries a predominant position. It may not be immediately obvious, and it rarely reveals itself in the first session. It takes time, often weeks, before the texture of their stance becomes clear. The work is less about ticking diagnostic markers and more about noticing the quality of contact, the silences, the urgency, the guilt, the withdrawal.

The phrases I offer in the chapters ahead are not scripts but fragments of language I have found useful in practice. Some can be used across therapies, but their potency increases when aligned with the position the young person inhabits.

While the vignettes are fictionalised to protect confidentiality, they are drawn directly from real cases. Every individual whose story informed them had received a formal OCD diagnosis and scored in the severe range on standardised measures. The details are altered, but the clinical reality is not.

This is not a replacement for ERP. Rather, when the position has been identified and a therapeutic alliance established, ERP can often be returned to in a way that feels more bearable and effective. The greatest successes come when structured exposure is integrated with, not substituted for, an appreciation of the psychic position.

For clinicians, this threshold requires tolerance of uncertainty. It means resisting the urge to rush toward symptom reduction when the atmosphere of the room tells a different story. Sometimes the most powerful intervention is to wait until the position declares itself.

What begins in these small shifts of attention becomes the map for everything that follows. From this foundation, the four positions can be heard as movements of mind rather than categories of diagnosis textures of being that reveal how the adolescent is managing their internal world.

Toward the Claustrum

The chapters that follow introduce four positions often encountered in adolescent OCD: the claustrum, the psychic retreat, the paranoid–schizoid, and the depressive. Each carries its own emotional atmosphere, its own way of organising thought, fear, and compulsion. They are not diagnostic categories but living stances, felt in the room through tone, silence, urgency, or guilt.

We begin with the claustrum, perhaps the most challenging to sit with. Here, the young person withdraws into a sealed psychic space, shutting out contact even while physically present. It is a position that tests the patience and endurance of any clinician, requiring tolerance of long stretches of silence, absence, and apparent inaccessibility.

To make these ideas more usable in practice, each chapter includes a call-out box. These are not substitutes for the full discussion, but anchors for busy clinicians – quick reminders of the texture of a position, common pit-falls, and ways of orienting therapeutic work. They are intended as guides to carry into the consulting room, while the deeper narrative remains in the chapters themselves.

The threshold is now crossed. What lies ahead are the positions them-selves – the psychic ground on which ERP, psychoanalytic work, or integrative practice must stand if they are to hold weight.

References

Bion, W. R. (1962). *Learning from experience.* London: Heinemann.

Fatori, D., Polanczyk, G. V., de Morais, R. M. C. B., & Asbahr, F. R. (2020). Long-term outcome of children and adolescents with obsessive–compulsive disorder: A 7–9-year follow-up of a randomized clinical trial. *European Child & Adolescent Psychiatry*, 29(11), 1613–1616. doi:10.1007/s00787-019-01457-8.

The Claustrum Position in OCD

Claustrum in Latin means an enclosure, a locked space. Erik Erikson has been acknowledged as introducing the metaphor in 1937 to describe the child's inner world as a prison (Willoughby, 2001). Half a century later, Donald Meltzer gave the idea its most detailed psychoanalytic form in *The Claustrum* (1992). For Meltzer, the claustrum was not stubbornness or resistance, but a genuine psychic position: a retreat into a sealed mental chamber that, though costly, offered safety against unbearable internal danger. He observed this most vividly in children and adolescents who struggled to meet ordinary therapy, and his insight remains clinically vital today.

Meltzer developed a very comprehensive model of the claustrum, describing different internal chambers that reflected how a young person experiences their relationship with the mother. It is a complex and imaginative theory, rich with detail. For the purpose of this book, I will not attempt to reproduce those technical intricacies. My aim is narrower: to show how even a simplified understanding of the claustrum offers a valuable way of working with adolescents whose obsessive-compulsive disorder (OCD) takes this shape. Readers who wish to pursue the deeper and more advanced aspects should turn to Meltzer's original text.

It is difficult to capture in words what such a position feels like. Clinically, however, the atmosphere in the room is unmistakable. I remember a 16-year-old girl who, after several sessions of near silence and minimal verbal exchange, finally whispered: 'If I let the thought out, it will break me inside.' Her voice was flat, her eyes fixed on the floor. She was not simply shy or reluctant to attend; she was locked in. The stillness was suffocating, as though even the smallest curiosity about her ritual might rupture something fragile. I found myself hesitating to ask even the most ordinary questions, how much time the ritual consumed, what it involved, because the room did not feel delicate, like walking on eggshells, but fortified, as if I were speaking to a mind that allowed almost nothing in and gave almost nothing out. That is the claustrum, not defiance, but psychic survival in a chamber of the mind.

Adolescence brings a sudden flood of sexual and aggressive impulses that can ignite claustral withdrawal. What overwhelms is not simply the existence

DOI: 10.4324/9781003729716-8

of desire, but its intensity, unpredictability, and the moral dilemmas it awakens. A fleeting image of arousal or a surge of anger may be felt as alien, even dangerous, as though the self is being invaded. In this position, the adolescent seeks safety not in thought or feeling but in control: objects ordered, taps repeated, actions rehearsed. Compulsions here function as a seal against inner life, a way of holding sexuality and aggression at bay. From the outside, the rituals look mechanical, even pointless, but internally they preserve psychic survival, keeping volatile impulses from breaking through and overwhelming the adolescent's fragile sense of self.

An adolescent overwhelmed by sudden anger or shame may retreat into counting rituals or silent mental rehearsals. The logic is inward: not to protect others, but to shield themselves from feelings that threaten to erupt. Each repetition functions like a lock on the door, layering protection against the unbearable.

Such compulsions – symmetry rituals, tapping, counting, ordering – are not habits. They are psychic glue, binding the adolescent at the seams at the very moment they fear emotional collapse. Without them, it can feel as if the self might disintegrate altogether.

From a clinical standpoint, the claustrum is not resistance but survival. The rigid, repetitive surface hides a fragile effort to manage unmanageable states of mind. Recognising this spares the clinician from miscasting the adolescent as oppositional, and instead allows a stance that is compassionate and developmentally attuned. When rituals serve a claustral function, they are not just symptoms to extinguish but lifelines holding overwhelming feelings at bay. Clinical work must approach them with care, not blunt eradication.

The claustrum is not only a defensive posture. It is a place. For the adolescent, it can feel safe and stifling but also protective and imprisoning. Obsessions and compulsions provide the structure of this inner space, holding it together and keeping the outside world at bay. This is the inner world to which we now turn.

Conceptual Overview – The Inner World of the Claustrum

While the claustrum can be described as a defensive retreat against overwhelming thoughts and feelings, its inner reality is more complex and more tragic. Donald Meltzer (1992) reminds us that the claustrum is not only a barrier against danger but an entire way of living inside the mind, built from fear, fantasy, and fragmentation. For the young person caught there, it becomes both life-support and prison. I often think of it as a womb and a tomb. A womb because it can feel safe, warm, and cut off from the pressures of both the outside world and the inner world. A tomb because, over time, it becomes airless and restrictive, preventing emotional growth and leaving the adolescent sealed away and out of reach. Sorensen (2016) makes a similar point, describing the claustrum as a psychic space that begins as safety but eventually drains vitality, leaving the young person cut off from real connection.

Inside this state, the adolescent is not merely shielding themselves from pain. They are struggling to control what feels like an internal catastrophe, fearing that direct contact with grief, rage, shame or longing would cause them to break apart. Omnipotent rituals and fantasies of control take the place of real relationships. For adolescents who reside in a claustral position in relation to their OCD, compulsions appear as facts. They do not negotiate with them. They simply act as though the logic were airtight. Even curiosity about the ritual can drive them further inward, sometimes to the point of leaving therapy altogether. Repetition, whether phrases, checking, or ordering, keeps unbearable emotions locked away. The protection comes at a cost of loneliness, rigidity, and slowed emotional growth.

The claustrophobic quality of this defence is hard to overstate. The longer a young person remains within it, the more alien and unsafe the outside world feels. Even small signs of genuine feeling, a sigh, a flicker of anger, or a collapse of certainty, can provoke terror or shame. The claustrum convinces the adolescent that survival depends on maintaining this sealed-off world at any cost.

Recent qualitative research with Tavistock-trained child psychotherapists (Veiga, 2021) supports this framing. In a doctoral study exploring clinical uses of the claustrum concept, therapists described young people who appeared sealed off, unreachable, and ritualised. These adolescents were not simply resistant or oppositional, they were psychically fortified. In the countertransference, therapists reported feelings of stuckness, exclusion, and suffocation. The clinical picture closely mirrors what is described here. Compulsions functioned not as negotiable behaviours but as the non-negotiable logic of psychic survival. Though unpublished, the thesis strengthens the view of the claustrum as more than metaphor and as a working clinical position that remains deeply relevant in adolescent practice.

For the clinician, grasping the inner reality of the claustrum is essential. Without it, there is a risk of underestimating the depth of retreat, imagining it as simple avoidance rather than a desperate form of preservation. Interventions aimed at dismantling defences may be felt as catastrophic betrayals. Emerging from the claustrum is not about compliance or sudden insight. It is a profound risk that requires new foundations of trust, containment, and resilience. Sorensen (2016) reminds us that claustral states can be understood on a continuum, from everyday moments of entrapment to severe psychic imprisonment. The adolescents described in the clinical examples that follow sit at the more entrenched end of this spectrum, where compulsions function as airtight facts and claustral retreat becomes central to their OCD.

When an adolescent resides in this position, they often feel deeply unreachable, making emotional or therapeutic contact difficult. In the chapters that follow, the four positions will be shown as the central way of understanding intrusive thoughts and compulsions. Here, with the claustrum, the clinical examples and transcripts illustrate how this psychic position shapes OCD. Recognising when a young person is caught in the claustrum is not optional but essential. Many adolescents will return again and again to this tight internal space, and without this framework their struggles risk being misread as resistance, non-compliance, or even treatment failure.

I recall a 15-year-old boy who spent hours each evening tapping the corners of his desk in a precise sequence before he could attempt sleep. When I asked what would happen if he did not complete this sequence, he did not offer the usual explanations about harm coming to family or disasters occurring. He simply said, 'I can't not do it.' His tone was flat, final, and without curiosity. To him, the ritual was not a belief to be questioned but a fact to be obeyed. When I suggested trying to delay the tapping by even a few seconds, he closed down and stared at the floor, as if I had threatened to undo the very structure holding him together. In that moment, it was clear that the ritual was not about avoiding catastrophe in the outside world, but about preventing collapse inside.

In my countertransference I noticed my own thinking stall, accompanied by a felt tightness. It seemed as though there were no entrances and no exits, no way into the boy's mind and no way out. What struck me was that this stalling did not carry the familiar anxieties clinicians know well, such as fears of incompetence or of not being good enough. Instead, it had a different quality, almost airless. There was no urge to be inventive or creative, no impulse to try a clever intervention. On some level, I knew any such attempt would simply fall flat. This is the lived atmosphere of the claustrum in the clinic, a fortified inner chamber where compulsions hold the adolescent together but at the cost of shutting out emotional contact.

The clinical vignettes that follow illustrate a pattern described in detail below: an inward pull, emotional flattening, withdrawal from relationship, and rituals lived as residence rather than protection.

Clinical Examples of the Claustrum Position in OCD

Jack

Jack, a 15-year-old boy, was referred by his general practitioner (GP) with a query of severe OCD due to his struggles with unwanted intrusive thoughts. In the first session, he was polite and cooperative but engaged only on a surface level. At first, this was attributed to adolescent awkwardness and the hesitancy of a first meeting.

As the sessions unfolded, a clear pattern emerged. Jack described compulsions around symmetry, driven by an overwhelming need for things to feel 'right'. When asked what might happen if he resisted the compulsions, his answers were vague. 'Nothing. I just wouldn't feel right'. He denied contamination fears, worries about harm, or fear of failure. His rituals were not about warding off an external danger but about restoring an internal sense of balance.

From the clinician's perspective, the countertransference was striking. There was a persistent sense of frustration and restlessness, an urge to push harder and shake something loose. Yet every effort seemed to thicken the wall between them. At times, the clinician felt flattened, their own emotional tone mirroring Jack's.

Jack illustrates the claustral dynamic: no external object, rituals as residence, emotional flatness, and the projection of stasis into the therapeutic relationship. Recognising this helped reframe his apparent 'non-engagement' not as resistance but as evidence of the claustral position itself.

Sarah

Sarah, a 17-year-old student, was referred after her teachers noticed her compulsive urge to tap objects during lessons. She would stop her work to tap wooden surfaces several times, disrupting her learning and distracting others. At home, her parents saw the same behaviour and worried about its effect on her daily life.

When asked about her rituals, Sarah shrugged. 'I don't know. It just doesn't feel right otherwise.' She denied anxiety and insisted the only drawback was the time it consumed. Despite her parents' concern, she resisted exploration of feelings, offering flat replies such as 'fine' or 'I guess so.'

In sessions, the atmosphere was one of lifelessness. Questions were often met with the same blank responses:

THERAPIST: What happens if you don't tap?
SARAH: Nothing. I just can't move on until I do.
THERAPIST: How does it feel once it's done?
SARAH: It's just done. I can carry on.

Whenever the therapist attempted behavioural experiments, Sarah appeared superficially cooperative but remained emotionally disengaged. The countertransference was one of futility, as though nothing could land. At times, the therapist noticed themselves trying harder and harder, as if testing locked doors one after another while Sarah stayed motionless. Eventually, Sarah described herself as 'numb' and 'invisible'. This seemed to capture not only her inner state but also the therapeutic relationship itself.

Jack and Sarah together show two faces of the claustrum. Jack demonstrates the inward pull toward symmetry rituals with no external object, while Sarah reveals the flatness and relational withdrawal that leave the therapist feeling invisible. In both, the rituals are not simply behaviours but lifelines of psychic survival.

Clinical Transcripts

Jack

THERAPIST: Can you tell me what happens if the books on your desk are not
lined up exactly?
JACK: I just cannot leave it like that.

(Annotation: A flat statement of fact. No fear of harm is given, only an
inward compulsion to act.)

THERAPIST: What do you think would happen if you did leave them?
JACK: Nothing. It would just feel wrong.

(Annotation: No external danger is invoked. The language centres on
feeling 'wrong' and points inward rather than outward.)

THERAPIST: And how do you feel when everything is lined up?
JACK: It is fine then. I do not think about it.

(Annotation: The ritual restores temporary balance but brings no sense of
relief. The therapist may feel deflated by the lack of affect.)

THERAPIST: Do you ever wonder why it has to feel exactly right?
JACK: I do not know. It just does.

(Annotation: Shrugs and short replies close down symbolic exploration.
The atmosphere is one of stasis, leaving the therapist circling in place.)

Sarah's early sessions were marked by minimal responses and a detached
tone. Her rituals of tapping were described without affect, as if they were
simple facts of life. Attempts to introduce imagination or explore emotional
meaning were met with silence or brief shrugs. I often felt myself over-
working, trying to generate dialogue while she remained still and disengaged.
The sense of futility in the room was palpable. The transcript below
illustrates this quality of stuckness in the early encounters.

Sarah

THERAPIST: Sarah, your parents mentioned that you have been doing a lot of
counting lately. Can you tell me what it is like for you when you do that?
SARAH: (shrugs): I just do it. It is not really a big deal.

(Annotation: Her shrug and flat tone gave me the immediate sense of being
pushed to the edges. I felt peripheral, as though my question had no weight.)

THERAPIST: It sounds like it is taking up a lot of your time. What happens if you do not count?

SARAH: (flat tone): It just does not feel right. I do not know how to explain it. I cannot move on until I do it.

(Annotation: No catastrophe is named. The focus is on an internal state of 'rightness'. I wanted to help her articulate more, yet nothing seemed to open. The atmosphere tightened.)

THERAPIST: What do you think would happen if you did not finish counting to 200?

SARAH: (pauses, looks uncomfortable): I do not think anything would happen. I just would not be able to stop thinking about it. It would feel wrong.

(Annotation: For a moment, the pause made me hopeful that reflection was coming. But her answer circled back into flatness. The sense of futility returned. Nothing could move forward.)

THERAPIST: So the counting helps you feel better in a way?

SARAH: I guess. It just makes things even. Balanced. (Looks away and picks at her fingernail.)

(Annotation: 'Balance' is presented as a fact, not a feeling. Her turning away and fiddling left me disconnected. My words seemed to slide off her, unreceived.)

THERAPIST: Do you ever think about why you need things to feel balanced?

SARAH: (shrugs): Not really. I have always been like this.

(Annotation: Another shrug, another closure. I noticed myself becoming unusually active, tempted to keep pushing with new angles, as if trying locked doors one after another. Each one shut immediately.)

THERAPIST: How do you feel when you finish counting? Does it make you calm or happy?

SARAH: (flatly): Not really. It is just done. I can move on.

(Annotation: The ritual did not relieve or soothe. It simply allowed continuation. I felt drained, my own energy mirroring the lifelessness of the exchange.)

THERAPIST: That sounds exhausting. Does it bother you to count so much?

SARAH: (pauses): I do not know. I just do it. It is not worth thinking about.

(Annotation: This final line captured the claustral feel most starkly. Thought was shut down before it could begin. The session flattened out, as though vitality had been drained from the room.)

Commentary

Jack and Sarah show different faces of the claustrum. Jack illustrates the compulsion toward symmetry with no external object, while Sarah demonstrates the deadened atmosphere of repetition and disengagement. In both, the defining feature is not the ritual itself but the stance toward it: flat, inwardly focused, and resistant to symbolic elaboration. For the clinician, the countertransference – whether restlessness, futility, or a creeping sense of invisibility – often reveals as much as the adolescent's words. Together, these examples show how the claustrum is recognised less by content than by the atmosphere it creates in the room.

How the Claustrum Appears in the Room

The exchanges with Jack and Sarah illustrate how different surface behaviours can point to the same underlying stance. What unites them is not the form of their compulsions but the atmosphere they create, which is flat, inwardly focused, and resistant to elaboration. As therapists, we often feel this as restlessness, futility, or even invisibility, the sense that our words cannot land. To make sense of this recurring pattern, I have described five hallmarks that together form the profile of the claustrum position. These are not rules or a checklist but recurring textures in the room that, when seen together, bring the claustrum into view.

An Absent or Empty External Object

In the claustrum, fear or anxiety is often turned inward and lacks a meaningful external reference point. Unlike more familiar forms of OCD, where fears may centre on contamination or harm to others, the adolescent's rituals serve primarily to manage an internal sense of imbalance or discomfort.

At times, the external object seems absent altogether. At other times, it is present but hollow, mentioned without emotional weight or elaboration. For example, an adolescent may say that 'something bad' might happen if they resist a ritual, but they struggle to specify what that bad thing is, or they describe it in flat, affectless terms. The object is there in language but stripped of symbolic life.

Instead, their expressions circle around restoring a subjective sense of rightness. Adolescents often say, 'It just feels right,' 'I just feel like I need to,' or 'It will not feel right if I don't.' In this way, the ritual functions less to neutralise a feared event in the outside world and more to shore up an internal sense of stability.

These phrases reflect the drive to restore internal balance rather than neutralise an external threat. A young person may spend hours aligning items on a desk, not from fear that misalignment will cause harm, but to alleviate an undefined inner tension.

It is important to note that feelings of rightness on their own do does not confirm the claustrum position. Many adolescents with OCD describe this phenomenon. At times, silence or brief replies may reflect something different, such as shame, fear of embarrassment, or anxiety about revealing a feared thought. In such cases, cutting down conversation functions as a defence against exposure rather than as evidence of the claustral stance. It is only when a therapeutic relationship is established and the adolescent continues to describe rituals without a clear external threat that this feature more reliably points to the claustrum. What matters is not a single marker but the convergence of this inward focus with the other features that together make up the claustral profile.

Emotional Flattening or Disconnection

Adolescents in a claustrum position often present with a muted emotional tone and a sense of being walled off. They may describe long hours of ritual with the same tone they use to recount what they had for lunch or what they did at school. Conversations feel strangely flat, as if something vital is missing.

For example:

THERAPIST: How do you feel when it is finished?
ADOLESCENT: It is just done.
THERAPIST: And what happens if you do not do it?
ADOLESCENT: Nothing really. I just have to.

The sense is not of resistance but of absence. In the room, therapists often feel blocked or paralysed, as though their words cannot land. Meltzer described this atmosphere in his original work on the claustrum as a walled-off psychic chamber, and the countertransference often reflects this.

It is important to note that withdrawal and flatness are common in adolescence. At times, they reflect ordinary self-protection or they can arise in the context of trauma. Services must always remain trauma informed, asking whether apparent flatness may be dissociation or numbing. What marks the claustrum is the consistency of the disconnection, especially when it intensifies whenever talk turns toward rituals and intrusive thoughts.

Absence of Symbolic Play

The claustrum forecloses imagination. Thoughts are not treated as symbols that can be explored, but as raw facts to be endured. When invited to reflect, the adolescent tends to give short, literal replies:

THERAPIST: What do you think the ritual helps with?
ADOLESCENT: Nothing. I just do it.

THERAPIST: If you stopped?
ADOLESCENT: It would not feel right. That is all.

Attempts to invite imaginative openings quickly close down. If asked to turn a thought into a story, or draw it as an image, the adolescent may respond, 'It is just a thought,' or, 'There is nothing to draw.' Pictures, if produced, are neat but empty. Stories are repetitive and stripped of symbolic content.

Of course, imagination varies across young people. Neurodiversity, developmental stage, and personality style all shape how symbolic play appears in therapy. A limited imaginative range does not by itself signal the claustrum. What matters is the combination of literalness with the other features of the claustral stance, especially inward focus and psychic stasis.

From the therapist's side, the countertransference often includes a sense of futility or boredom. I have noticed myself becoming unusually active, asking more questions, trying new approaches, almost as if testing one locked door after another. When each door shuts immediately, it signals that symbolic play has been foreclosed. This is not resistance in the usual sense, but an enclosure where thoughts are lived as brute facts rather than shared symbols.

Withdrawal from Relationship

In the claustrum position, adolescents often retreat from live connection with others. They may attend sessions but remain emotionally absent, their rituals serving as a barrier that quietly excludes the therapist. The atmosphere is not one of hostility or defiance, but of distance, as if relationship has no real value.

For example:

THERAPIST: Can I sit with you in how hard this feels?
ADOLESCENT: You do not need to.
THERAPIST: Would you like me to understand what it is like?
ADOLESCENT: (Shrugs, turns away): It does not matter.

The withdrawal does not feel oppositional. It is not the adolescent pushing back against intrusion, but rather a stance of indifference, as though interpersonal contact has been quietly set aside. At times, the compulsion itself functions as a shield: a young person may count under their breath or fiddle with shoelaces while questions are asked, signalling a preference for ritual over relationship.

In the countertransference, the therapist may feel oddly invisible, as if their presence hardly registers. Their words slide off as though there is no receiver. This sense of futility or irrelevance is a powerful marker of the claustrum atmosphere.

It is important to remember that withdrawal is also common in depression, social anxiety, or simply in the ordinary turbulence of adolescence.

What makes it claustral is the consistency of this stance and its convergence with the other hallmarks, especially inward focus and absence of symbolic play.

Stasis and Avoidance of Ambivalence

Adolescents with OCD often struggle to manage conflicting feelings, but in the claustrum this difficulty becomes defining. Love and anger toward a parent, for example, cannot be held together. One state of mind must be sealed off or the whole structure feels at risk of collapse.

This creates a sense of stasis. Moments that could invite development – thinking about a relationship, reflecting on a choice, exploring a new idea – are quickly shut down. Rituals step in to provide false certainty. A fleeting glimpse of ambivalence is often followed by a tightening of compulsive behaviours.

THERAPIST: Can you feel both proud and worried about what you did?
ADOLESCENT: No. It is just wrong.
THERAPIST: Could it be a bit of both?
ADOLESCENT: That does not make sense. It has to be one.

When I tentatively highlight ambivalence or suggest alternative possibilities, the response is rarely, 'I see what you mean, but it is difficult.' More often, it is silence, a turning away, or a refusal to contemplate. The very idea of ambivalence seems warded off before it can be considered.

In countertransference, the quality is one of heaviness or suspension, as if time itself has stalled. Nothing seems to move forward, because conflict cannot be borne. Unlike oppositionality, this does not feel like attack. It feels more like disengagement, as if the adolescent is no longer engaged in the project of growth.

Difficulty with ambivalence can be found across adolescence and in many mental health conditions. What marks the claustrum is the pervasive atmosphere of halted development, where the avoidance of ambivalence produces psychic stasis and freezes the therapeutic encounter.

Summary

Taken together, these five hallmarks form the profile of the claustrum position. No single feature in isolation is decisive, but when they converge, the pattern is clear: an inward focus without external object, rituals lived as residence, the absence of symbolic play, withdrawal from relationship, and suspension of growth through the avoidance of ambivalence.

What distinguishes the claustrum is not the content of obsessions or compulsions but the stance toward them. Rituals are not used to neutralise an external danger but to create a sealed chamber in which the adolescent lives.

Thoughts are not explored as symbols but endured as facts. Relationship is not attacked but set aside, leaving the therapist to feel restless, futile, or invisible.

For clinicians, recognising this pattern is less about diagnosis and more about orientation. It reminds us to attune to the atmosphere in the room, to notice what is stirred in our own countertransference, and to observe how the adolescent relates to their own mind. When these textures are present, interventions need to be slowed, softened, and grounded in containment.

> ### Box 8.1 Recognising the Claustrum
>
> - The atmosphere feels airless or stalled, as though time has slowed.
> - Affect is flat or narrowed; the adolescent may speak in brief, literal statements.
> - Rituals are described as facts ('I just have to') rather than as protection against catastrophe.
> - Odd compliance may occur: the adolescent appears cooperative but with little curiosity or engagement.
> - Countertransference often includes suffocation, futility, or the urge to overwork.
> - Contact with sexual or aggressive feeling is avoided; moral conflict is sealed of from conscious thought.

Working Clinically

Working with adolescents in a claustrum position is demanding and emotionally taxing. One reason some young people are prematurely discharged as non-engaging or 'not ready' may be that they are operating from this stance. In time-limited services where quick results are expected, it can feel as if the war is lost before the battle begins.

Some adolescents in a claustrum position can eventually engage in exposure and response prevention (ERP). If ERP is hurried or forced, however, claustral defences harden. The work that follows is not a set of steps. It is a stance. These approaches help us meet the adolescent at the walls of the enclosure without forcing entry, and stay steady enough for small cracks of contact to appear in their own time.

Holding the Atmosphere

The clinician needs to tolerate being perceived as intrusive or persecutory without taking that perception as truth. At times, you may feel simply not right for the young person. The chemistry can feel off and it can seem as if you did not connect. That experience can be valid in other contexts, yet in the claustrum almost anything said can be felt as intrusive or persecutory. If the adolescent keeps turning up, treat that continuity as the key signal at first.

We bear projected anxiety, criticism, and mistrust without retaliating, without collapsing into defensiveness and without withdrawing. The room may feel charged with suspicion or silent hostility. These are reflections of the adolescent's internal world, not reliable readings of the relationship. Regular supervision or reflective practice is essential. These feelings can stir emotional turmoil and can nudge clinicians into decisions that do not match their usual style, for example pushing the pace, changing approach abruptly, or pronouncing the young person unmotivated.

Language matters. Statements about motivation or interest need to be used carefully and compassionately. They should not become a defensive move. Service pressure can make the wish to move claustrum cases along very strong, especially when other recent cases have been livelier. Naming that pressure in supervision helps contain it and protects the work.

By staying present, we model something new. Being seen, questioned, or mistrusted does not have to end in abandonment or attack. While past events matter, hunting for a historical explanation too early can become a red herring. The focus stays with the live encounter.

Naming the Position

We can acknowledge the stance explicitly, without attacking or colluding with it. Gentle, ordinary language works best:

> It seems hard to be here, but you still come. That tells me this space matters, even if we do not yet know how.
> I get the sense that talking feels risky. We can go at a pace that works for you.
> Sometimes it feels safer to stay in your own head than to be here with me. I wonder if that feels true?

Such remarks keep the position in view. They contrast with what many young people hear elsewhere, which is to 'snap out of it'. Naming the stance honours the truth of their position and shows it can be thought about rather than simply obeyed. In effect, what we are saying is: I know you are here, I know it is hard, and I am not going to keep poking at you until you talk. I will not tell you off or tell your parents that you are not engaging. I will keep naming how stuck it feels and how hard it is for you. My words may feel intrusive or persecutory at first, but if I can hold steady in that atmosphere, the space gradually becomes safer to inhabit together.

I recall a 14-year-old boy for whom even taking out his AirPods felt impossible. His mother, frustrated, insisted he remove them before leaving us to begin the session. He looked at me briefly, then at the floor, as if testing whether I would criticise him for being rude or unmotivated. I simply named what seemed true: that it must feel more comfortable and safe with the

AirPods in, that they offered a concrete way of blocking out my words, and that not having them made it harder. Nothing shifted for weeks. Then, one session, he smirked as his hand went to his pocket where the AirPods were tucked away. I commented that perhaps something I had said felt dangerous and he was tempted to shut me out. The smirk seemed like a moment of recognition: a silent admission that yes, part of him wanted to hide completely. It was not a dramatic breakthrough, but it was a shared naming of his stance. That acknowledgement, not condemnation, not pressure, marked the first small loosening of the claustral walls.

Softening the Demand for Engagement

Pressure tends to tighten the retreat. I picture the adolescent gripping something that feels precious and safe. The more we ask for it, the tighter the grip. Our task is to make loosening feel possible without demands.

> You do not have to say anything right now. We can sit together and see what comes.
> You do not have to answer. I wonder if part of you wants to be here and another part does not.
> There is no rush. Having someone alongside you can be enough.
> It is okay if talking feels difficult today. We can think together about why.

In many clinical contexts, this stance allows shy, reluctant, or traumatised adolescents to settle. Given time, sessions often take on a more natural shape, with conversation gradually emerging. With adolescents in the claustrum, however, the process is different. The same reassurances need to be repeated, often again and again. I may begin with a comment about a ritual, receive only a brief or closed response, then notice the adolescent's anxiety rise as if my curiosity itself were persecutory. At such moments, I soften the encounter by naming how difficult it feels and by making clear that there is no demand.

This pattern can go on for many weeks, and sometimes months. Yet, it is worthwhile. When the grip eventually loosens, even slightly, more aspects of the person can come into the room. What begins to emerge then is not just more speech, but more insight into the function of the OCD and the protective role of the claustrum itself.

Using Metaphor to Encourage Symbolic Thinking

Symbolic language can sometimes help when direct description fails. If used too soon, however, it can prompt withdrawal. I tend to introduce metaphor only later, once containment and safety have been established in the room.

It can feel like being in a room with no doors. I wonder if there is a window anywhere?
Some people describe their thoughts as a maze. I wonder what yours feel like?
If this feeling were a character, what would it be like?
Imagine your thoughts as a room. What is inside? What is locked away?

Metaphor is invited, not imposed. When the timing is right, imagery becomes a bridge between the sealed interior and a shared language.

In my experience, symbolic play is often almost absent in the claustrum. I recall an adolescent who had been with me for 39 sessions, a young man I had nearly given up on by session six because everything was so shut down and intense. By this stage, I had immersed myself in the claustrum literature and was beginning to think differently about his relationship with OCD. A metaphor came to mind, one I believe originated with Meltzer or from his group supervisions: that he was both the prison officer and the prisoner of his OCD. For reasons that surprised us both, this image connected deeply with him. From that point onward, we returned to the metaphor every week.

As his symptoms eased, our conversations extended into what it must feel like for a prisoner to leave confinement, the fear of losing structure and routine, and the relief of freedom. By session 45 we were able to begin ERP experiments, and by session 60 he was well enough to be discharged. At review, three months later, he was a new person: animated, studying, working a part-time job. It was an incredibly positive outcome. That metaphor, which seemed to shift the work, remains etched in my mind.

Gently Exploring the Function of the Claustrum

The claustrum protects. Naming its function validates the dilemma. The retreat keeps something unbearable at bay, but it has a cost. We explore the function first, then the cost.

I wonder if keeping things the same feels safer than the risk of change?
If you did not have to be so sure, what do you imagine might happen?
It seems that the unknown brings up a lot. Maybe the patterns help you keep control.
Sometimes being in our own world feels like the only way to stay safe. Is there a way to be safe and connected at the same time?

This stance is not a probe to break down defences. It is recognition. Often, the adolescent has never heard their retreat described in this way. To have it named as protective, rather than as laziness or lack of motivation, can be disarming. At times, the simple acknowledgement brings a flicker of response, a pause, a glance, or a slight softening in the room. These are the first hairline cracks in the wall.

In most therapies, the sequence is familiar: we name the defence, highlight its function to lessen shame or guilt, and then turn gently to its cost. In the claustrum, the process is slower and more layered. We begin by tolerating being perceived as intrusive, by naming the atmosphere itself, and by showing that we can sit alongside the position without retreating or retaliating. Only after this ground has been established do we move carefully from naming the function into considering its cost.

Speaking through Story

Metaphor can sometimes be taken further by placing the adolescent's experience into the frame of a story. Rather than naming their position directly, the therapist introduces a third figure, image, or character. This creates distance and reduces shame. The adolescent is not being asked to explain themselves but to notice something about a story told together.

> It is like living in a castle you built yourself. It is strong and it is lonely. Imagine a story where someone is lost in a maze and cannot find the way out. I wonder what you notice.

Earlier, I described using the image of being both the prison officer and the prisoner of OCD. That metaphor became a shared language for one young man and allowed us, over time, to explore what it felt like to face freedom after confinement. Speaking through story develops this approach further. It allows us to explore claustral states without confronting the adolescent head-on, which can so easily feel persecutory.

These are invitations, not interpretations. If the adolescent adds even a small detail, it is a sign that the walls are not absolute. My own imagination can be a useful guide here. If I find myself picturing caves, castles, or exile, I may share these images gently and tentatively, if the timing feels safe. Sometimes the adolescent simply listens. At other times, they offer a word or a gesture of recognition. Even that small response can shift the atmosphere, suggesting that symbolic language has begun to re-enter the room.

I recall working with a girl who had been largely silent for weeks. Knowing she had loved the outdoors as a child, I tentatively said, 'It is a little like being in a tree house with no ladder. You are safe up there, but cut off.' She looked at me, smirked, and replied, 'That would be fine, as long as I had Netflix.' It was only a brief moment, but it mattered. The story gave her a way to acknowledge her position indirectly, with humour and a touch of play. From then on, the tree house image became a shared reference point. It allowed us to think together about the safety of being enclosed, and the costs of being cut off, without her feeling pushed to speak about it directly.

Naming the Risk without Forcing Action

We can name the frightening choice without pushing movement. Both safety and growth carry risk.

> It makes sense that staying safe feels better than trying something new. Staying safe has a cost too, and only you can decide when it is time to risk it.

Holding back from urging change often softens the room. The young person feels seen rather than managed. Acknowledging the choice, without expectation, can create a small shift.

I recall a 13-year-old who had spent many sessions in silence. One day I said, 'It feels like we are just sitting with the silence.' She looked up and asked, 'Why?' The word itself put me on the spot, but what struck me was the emotion behind it. It was more alive than anything we had touched in the previous sessions. That moment reminded me that even the smallest exchange can signal movement. By naming the risk without pressing for change, space had opened for something new to emerge.

Modelling Non-persecutory Presence

In the claustrum, the presence of another person can be experienced as persecutory, while their absence can feel annihilating. The therapist's task is to offer a presence that is steady but not intrusive, engaged but not demanding.
Curiosity:

> I wonder what it feels like to imagine letting me see a little more. Not that you have to. I am curious what the idea feels like.

Silence:

> It feels like there is a lot you are holding silently. That is okay. We can sit with it together.

Both curiosity and silence are ways of modelling contact that does not persecute and does not abandon. Over time, this quality of steady, non-demanding presence can loosen the hold of the claustrum and make the room feel safer to inhabit.

I remember sitting with an adolescent who spent much of the session in silence, staring at the floor. I said, 'It feels like there is a lot you are holding quietly, and that is okay. We can sit with it together.' He did not speak, but after a long pause his shoulders dropped slightly and his breathing slowed. It was a tiny shift, but it felt like the room had softened. The moment reminded me that presence itself can be therapeutic, even when no words are exchanged.

When We Inevitably Misstep

Repair is a universal part of any therapeutic relationship. All clinicians move too fast at times, or miss a cue. With adolescents in a claustrum stance, these moments can feel more charged. A small misstep may be taken as proof of persecution or abandonment. At the same time, the therapist may feel frustrated, bored, or even irritated by the young person's apparent inactivity. Recognising those reactions is essential, so they do not slip into unacknowledged defensiveness.

The important thing is to name the moment openly and with care.

> I think I pushed that too fast. I want you to feel unpressured here.

Naming the misstep without defence shows that contact can survive errors. Rather than glossing over it or withdrawing, we acknowledge it. Often the wall feels a little less absolute afterward, and the adolescent begins to learn that a relationship can hold steady even when mistakes are made.

When Rules Become a Prison

Rigid mental rules often begin as protection against chaos and uncertainty. At first, they can feel like a fortress, strong and reliable. Over time, they harden into a prison. Our task is not to smash these structures but to create room for flexibility.

> I get the sense there is a right way to do things and if it is not exactly right, it does not count.
> Does it ever feel like your mind runs a set of rules you have to follow?
> What is the worst thing that might happen if you did not check that thought one more time?
> It seems very precise, almost like an internal system running in the background.

I recall a young person who, after many silent sessions, began to offer brief glimpses of her inner world. She told me her mind felt like a surveillance system, with cameras watching 24 hours a day. If she did not follow the rules, she believed something terrible would happen. This image captured the prison-like quality of her OCD more clearly than anything I could have put into words. It also gave us a way to think together about the cost of living under constant monitoring and the possibility of finding moments of freedom.

As clinicians, we may find ourselves pulled into matching this rigidity, becoming overly precise in our language, or else feeling the urge to rebel against it. Both countertransference pulls are informative. Naming the structure without shaming it validates its function and gently hints at its cost.

Supporting Small Experiments in Engagement

Small experiments are essential in claustrum work. These are not exposure exercises in the usual sense, and they are not tasks to be completed. They are tiny invitations that sit just beyond the current enclosure. The purpose is not to confront fear head-on but to test whether the rigid hold of the claustrum can be softened without overwhelming the adolescent.

> I wonder if we could try something small today, such as letting a thought be there without fixing it.
> What would happen if we paused before the ritual and noticed what the urge feels like?
> Maybe we can think about the tiniest step forward, not changing everything, just a little shift.
> We do not have to do anything big. Even noticing what it is like to consider change is a step.

These small experiments differ from structured ERP because the emphasis is not on habituation to anxiety but on creating a lived experience that change, however slight, can be survivable. Even a flicker of difference in the room – a pause before the ritual, a glance at the therapist, or a few words such as 'maybe things do not always have to be this way' – can signal that the claustrum's rigidity is loosening.

Impatience often stirs in me at this point. It is easy to long for bigger progress, faster. When I can hold that back and match the adolescent's pace, the smallest shifts take on real significance. Over time, these micro-experiments accumulate and prepare the ground for more direct work, including ERP, once the adolescent feels safe enough to risk it.

Exploring the Relationship with the Therapist

In most psychodynamic therapies, an essential feature is to bring the relationship with the clinician actively into the room. With adolescents in a claustrum position, this is not only useful but necessary. The default stance they place us in is one of persecution or intrusion. Unless we name and work with that dynamic, it is easy for the adolescent to withdraw further and for the therapy to stall.

The relationship is therefore a live place to explore engagement and withdrawal. The therapist may be experienced as another demand, another voice pressing in, or another figure to be shut out. Naming this gently can transform the frame.

> Sometimes I may feel like another person making demands. I wonder if that feels true.

I notice that when I ask a question there is a long pause. I am curious if answering feels risky.
I have a feeling that part of you wants to be understood and another part needs to stay hidden. Maybe we can make room for both.
I might be wrong, but I wonder if trusting me feels too much like letting me in.

These small acknowledgements show that the therapeutic relationship can bear mistrust, hesitation, and distance without collapsing. In claustrum work, that experience itself can be transformative. It offers the adolescent a new model of connection, one that does not persecute and does not abandon.

Engaging with Guilt and the Fear of Change

Guilt and fear of change are common in claustrum work. Any movement can feel like betrayal of the self, or an invitation to catastrophe. I often notice a heaviness when guilt enters the room, and I weigh words more carefully. That countertransference itself is a marker of the bind.

> Sometimes change feels like betraying the person you have always been. I wonder if that is true for you.
> If things were different, do you ever worry you would not feel like yourself?
> It sounds as though letting go might lead to something bad, inside or outside.
> Sometimes people keep going because they think they should. Maybe we can think about where the should comes from.

We name guilt and fear without challenging them head on. This makes change more thinkable and less frightening.

I recall a young person who, after months of careful work, whispered, 'If I stop, I won't be me anymore.' The statement was delivered flatly, but the weight behind it was clear. Rather than reassuring her that she would still be herself, I said, 'That makes sense. Letting go can feel like betraying the person you have always been.' She looked at me with tears in her eyes, then quickly turned away. Nothing more was said, but the moment lingered. It showed that guilt could be named and survived without collapse.

Making Space for Ambivalence

Ambivalence is central in the claustrum. The young person may long for change and fear it just as strongly. Our task is to hold both sides without rushing to resolve the conflict.

> It makes sense that part of you wants to change and another part does not. We can give both parts space here.

What if we do not choose between change and staying the same. What if we notice what both feel like.

Sometimes even talking about a problem makes it feel more real. I wonder if that is happening now.

It is okay to feel unsure. We can sit with that together.

When ambivalence can be borne in the room, uncertainty does not have to lead to collapse. The adolescent begins to see both the protective role of the claustrum and the costs of remaining inside it. Change starts to feel like evolution rather than betrayal.

I recall an adolescent who said, 'I want it gone, but I don't want it gone.' Rather than pushing for clarity, I replied, 'Both parts can have a place here.' He stared at me for a long time before quietly saying, 'That feels true.' It was a small shift, but the atmosphere changed. Holding the ambivalence together allowed us to think about the OCD without forcing resolution.

Closing Reflections on Interventions

Working clinically with the claustrum is slow, demanding, and at times disheartening. The techniques outlined here are less about technique in the narrow sense and more about posture: a way of standing at the walls without either attacking them or walking away. Across sessions, the common thread is a stance that names what is happening, validates its protective function, and gently makes space for something different. Change rarely arrives suddenly. It comes in flickers – a glance, a smirk, a pause before a ritual – and our task is to notice and stay steady with these small openings.

The adolescent does not live inside the claustrum alone. Parents and carers often feel confused, excluded, or pushed into unhelpful roles of nagging or withdrawal. The stance we take as clinicians has a parallel at home. Parents, too, need guidance on how to stay present without persecuting and how to step back without abandoning.

Guidance for Parents

(*For clinicians to use when communicating with families.*)

When I explain the claustrum to parents, I often say something like:

Sometimes your child retreats into an invisible psychological room. It is not something they do deliberately, and it is not laziness or defiance. It is a state of mind where they feel safest sticking to what is known and routine, avoiding the uncertainties of feelings, changes, or new experiences. For them it feels protective, even if from the outside it can look like shutting down.

Parents often describe their child in these moments as apathetic. They stop talking, resist change, avoid eye contact, or appear oddly compliant. These behaviours are easily misread as laziness or refusal. Clinicians can help parents reframe this: the retreat is not opposition; it is a way of shutting down feeling when it becomes too much.

What parents need to hear is that their role is not to argue their child out of it or to push with logic. The task is to stay close enough to be found, but not so close that the adolescent retreats further. Sometimes this means sitting quietly nearby. Sometimes it means keeping routines steady without adding new demands. Often it means tolerating silence without assuming rejection, which can be understandably emotionally isolating for the parents of the young person.

Simple gestures can be powerful. Leaving a cup of tea at the bedroom door, calmly saying 'I am here if you need me,' or simply being in the same room without pressure all communicate presence without intrusion. These acts give the young person space to test coming out of retreat without fear of being pushed too hard or left completely alone.

For many parents, this stance is counterintuitive. They feel a strong pull either to withdraw in frustration or to push harder in order to 'get through'. Both impulses are understandable. What matters is to hold steady in between, offering a presence that does not persecute and does not abandon.

Even when change feels painfully slow, it helps parents to know that their presence matters. By staying available without forcing, they show their child that relationships can be safe.

Summary and Clinical Take Home

The claustrum represents one of the most challenging psychic positions we encounter. Among the four positions, it is perhaps the hardest to work with because the atmosphere it creates, with its flatness, withdrawal, and stasis, can leave clinicians feeling stuck or defeated. This challenge is magnified in time-limited services where pressure to deliver quick results often collides with the slow, steady stance the claustrum requires.

In my clinical experience, the claustrum is relatively rare, but once recognised it is unmistakable. The young person often appears emotionally flat, engages only at a surface level, and presents with rituals that function as airtight facts. The countertransference mirrors this experience. We feel stuck, heavy, or shut out, as if trapped inside the adolescent's inner world. It is easy in these moments to misinterpret what is happening as defiance, non-engagement, or lack of motivation. In reality, the rituals and the atmosphere are protective structures, attempts to hold together a self that feels at risk of disintegration.

The key to working in this position is to hold hope while respecting the adolescent's airtight defences. Our task is not to dismantle the walls with force but to notice and gently expand the cracks that inevitably appear.

These openings may be only a pause, a glance, or a flicker of ambivalence, but they are footholds for change. Progress is slow, and sessions may feel draining, yet perseverance is essential. The aim is not to argue the adolescent out of their stance or to demand recognition of it, but to stand patiently outside the enclosure and signal through steadiness, containment, and time that survival does not have to mean isolation.

Where the claustrum disconnects from feeling, the psychic retreat negotiates with it, allowing selective contact when emotion feels safer.

Box 8.2 ERP and the Claustrum: When to Pause and When to Proceed

- Pause when the room stays flat and rituals tighten in response to curiosity.
- Build containment until small signs of symbolic life appear.
- Use micro experiments first to test tolerability.
- Begin ERP only once curiosity can be borne without claustral recoil.

Box 8.3 Clinician's Guidance to Parents

- Withdrawal is not defiance. Rituals often hold your child together rather than push you away.
- Keep daily routines steady and predictable.
- Reduce accommodation of rituals but avoid repeated reassurance.
- Notice and affirm small steps of contact, a glance, a question, or brief talk.
- Offer short, gentle invitations rather than pressing for closeness.
- Use plain, non-judgemental language: see rituals as survival attempts, not bad habits.

References

Meltzer, D. (1992). *The Claustrum: An investigation of claustrophobic phenomena.* Perthshire: Clunie Press.

Sorensen, P. B. (2016). Degrees of entrapment: living and dying in the claustrum. *Journal of Child Psychotherapy*, 42(1), 45–53. doi:10.1080/0075417X.2016.1140875.

Veiga, A. (2021) *Encounters in the Claustrum: An exploratory study of the Claustrum in contemporary psychoanalytic child and adolescent psychotherapy.* Professional Doctorate thesis, Tavistock and Portman NHS Foundation Trust/University of Essex.

Willoughby, R. (2001). The dungeon of thyself: The claustrum as pathological container. *International Forum of Psychoanalysis*, 10(2–3), 123–133. doi:10.1516/B53C-KLBD-KKWB-AN74.

Chapter 9

The Psychic Retreat Position in OCD

I find myself confused as Jessica sits opposite me in the consulting room. She is 15 and has lived with obsessive-compulsive disorder (OCD) that once took the form of contamination fears and handwashing rituals. Nothing unusual in itself. Yet. when she speaks with me, it is as if the OCD does not exist. She can be lively, articulate, even optimistic. But whenever our conversation approaches guilt or touches on conflict, she closes down. She turns away, changes the subject, or minimises the dispute. I know the issue is more emotionally charged than she allows into words. At those moments, the OCD seems to flare again, as if summoned by the very feelings she cannot bear to face. Between sessions, she may describe whole stretches of time when the thoughts and compulsions have gone quiet, and her parents report no obvious symptoms. Then, without warning, something stirs inside her and she retreats back into ritual. It is this pattern that defines the psychic retreat. This chapter explores what happens in those moments, what triggers this selective withdrawal, and why it so often shapes the lives of adolescents we see in our consulting rooms.

Conceptual Overview – The Nature of the Psychic Retreat

John Steiner (1993) described the psychic retreat as an internal refuge from unbearable emotional pain, a defensive shelter that secures safety only by stepping back from connection. In adolescents with OCD, this retreat does not usually appear as a collapse of functioning. By this I mean that, unlike the claustrum, it does not involve a complete shutdown of interaction or incoming experience. The young person may still attend school, complete tasks, and speak with ease, but beneath that appearance they have stepped back emotionally. It is a conditional withdrawal that emerges when the emotional temperature rises. A broad range of feelings can trigger it, including guilt, anger, envy, shame, and even excitement. At those moments, intrusive thoughts and compulsions often come to the fore. Unlike the claustrum, which functions like a permanent fortress, the retreat is pieced together temporarily. It is activated when emotion becomes intolerable, and dismantled again when calm returns.

DOI: 10.4324/9781003729716-9

This distinction is clinically important. In the claustrum, the adolescent seems cut off almost all the time, whatever the situation. In the psychic retreat, they may look lively and engaged when the emotional atmosphere is calm. Withdrawal occurs only when a feeling rises beyond what they can tolerate. It might be guilt, shame, anger, envy, or even excitement. At that point, intrusive thoughts and compulsions step forward, taking the place of emotional contact.

In practice, I have met many young people whose OCD seemed severe, yet they could describe stretches of time when the thoughts felt absent. It was only through the rhythm of therapy that the link became clear. The quiet periods coincided with moments of stability, when relational pressures had eased and difficult feelings were less stirred. The retreat did not mean the symptom had vanished. It meant the symptom was dormant, waiting until the next surge of emotional strain brought it forward again.

In therapy, these adolescents can be some of the most confusing to work with. On the surface, they seem fine. They are thoughtful, articulate, and often speak about their OCD with insight and apparent readiness for change. Yet, just as progress appears to gather shape, they withdraw. Sessions that once felt open and collaborative can become flat or avoidant, often without any clear reason. The sudden shift leaves the clinician uncertain whether something meaningful has happened or whether the ground has simply given way.

When explored carefully, these shifts almost always coincide with an emotionally provocative event. It might be an argument at home, a perceived moral failing, or a surge of anger, guilt, or envy that feels intolerable. For the clinician, this can be disorienting. The sense of progress drains away. What felt like a steady rhythm of work suddenly collapses, and the clinician is left chasing after someone who has slipped from view.

This is the essence of the psychic retreat. It is not a permanent fortress like the claustrum but a temporary sanctuary, pieced together when needed and dismantled when calm returns. The retreat is not always dramatic. It may appear as a spike in compulsions, a tightening of order, or a sudden over-investment in routine. However it looks, the function is the same. It shields the adolescent from feelings that feel too risky or destabilising to face directly.

These adolescents are often what I think of as stealth sufferers. On the surface, they appear thoughtful, articulate, even well adjusted. Teachers may praise them as diligent, peers describe them as easy company, and parents may feel reassured that their child is coping better than most. Yet this competence can be deceptive. Beneath the polish lies a fragile dependence on keeping certain feelings at bay. When guilt, anger, envy, shame, or even excitement press too close, the retreat is activated and symptoms step in. What looks like maturity is in fact a conditional stability, one that relies on avoidance rather than emotional contact.

It is perhaps not surprising that adolescence, with its flood of new emotions and impulses, can stir feelings that seem alien and unsettling. At these points, a young person may retreat into intrusive thoughts and compulsions, using them as a cover from experiences that feel too much to carry directly.

The following cases of two adolescents show how the psychic retreat takes shape in practice. Their stories highlight the subtle hallmarks of this position: engagement on the surface, but withdrawal the moment feelings threaten to break through.

Clinical Examples of the Psychic Position in OCD

Amira

Amira was 16, referred by her school's pastoral lead. She presented as articulate, diligent, and respectful. Her grades were excellent, and she was active in extracurricular activities. Teachers described her as a model student. Yet she had begun to experience what she called 'mental static': sudden waves of intrusive thoughts, mostly about contamination and moral failure.

In the first sessions, she spoke with poise and insight. She acknowledged her distress, described her compulsions clearly, and engaged well in formulation. Then, after a weekend disagreement with her mother about a long-buried family issue, she arrived distant, overly compliant, and emotionally flat. Her symptoms had spiked, yet she dismissed the change as 'just stress' and insisted it was nothing new.

When I tried to link the flare-up with family tension, she offered cognitive explanations. 'I just had too much revision.' 'I'm not sleeping well.' The shift was less in behaviour than in tone. She was there, yet not present. I noticed my own hope of progress draining, replaced by a sense of careful treading, as if the room itself had become fragile.

This pattern repeated across sessions. Whenever interpersonal or emotionally charged material surfaced, her functioning dipped just enough for symptoms to swell, while her outward self stayed high-performing. Over time, with steady work, Amira began to see her compulsions as a retreat from emotional vulnerability, especially from anger and disappointment. For her, these feelings were dangerous because they clashed with her image of being a good person.

Eli

Eli was 14, referred by her GP with a diagnosis of OCD. His rituals centred on checking locks and doors. In session, he was pleasant, talkative, and often humorous, downplaying his distress with comments such as, 'It's just something I do. Everyone has quirks.'

At first he described his rituals in a light, amused tone and deflected questions about feelings. When I asked what might happen if he did not check the locks, he replied, 'Maybe the house would get broken into, or something dumb like that.' The words were casual, but the atmosphere suggested something guarded beneath the humour.

After a falling out with his closest friend, Eli's symptoms spiked sharply. He began checking his bedroom door up to 30 times before bed. In session, he looked more tired but kept the same breezy, minimising tone. When I asked about the argument, he shrugged. 'It's not a big deal. People fall out all the time. It's normal.'

Sitting with him, I felt my own pull to match his lightness, to accept his words at face value, while also sensing something heavier beneath. It took several sessions of staying close without pressing before he could admit that he felt guilty, not for what was said, but for fearing he had disappointed his friend and could not repair the rupture. His checking became a retreat from that guilt, insulating him with ritual when closeness felt too risky.

Clinical Transcripts

Amira

THERAPIST: Last week you said the thoughts were much quieter. How was that for you?
AMIRA: It was fine. I didn't really notice them.

(Annotation: Calm and articulate. Symptoms described as if they simply disappeared. Tone suggests dismissal of deeper exploration.)

THERAPIST: And then you mentioned they came back over the weekend. What do you think made the difference?
AMIRA: I don't know. I had a lot of revision. Probably just stress.

(Annotation: Spike attributed to cognitive factors only. Emotional links avoided. I notice myself wanting to press harder, sensing something left unsaid.)

THERAPIST: Sometimes stress plays a part, yes. I wonder if anything else happened that might have made things harder.
AMIRA: (pauses, looks down): Not really. Nothing important.

(Annotation: A pause, then minimisation. She is present but not in contact. The withheld affect creates a sense of flatness.)

THERAPIST: I wonder if it felt difficult after the disagreement with your mum.

AMIRA: (smiles politely, shakes head): It's nothing. We're fine.

(Annotation: The retreat is clear here. A polite smile seals off emotion. I feel the session flatten, as if access has been quietly withdrawn.)

Eli

THERAPIST: Eli, how often are you checking the door these days?
ELI: Oh, loads. Probably 30 times before bed. It's kind of ridiculous, right? (smiles)

(Annotation: Humour and self-mockery. The ritual is acknowledged but lifted away from feeling. I catch myself smiling back, sensing I am colluding with the minimisation.)

THERAPIST: It sounds exhausting. What do you think makes it feel so important to check?
ELI: I don't know. Maybe burglars? Or maybe I just like being sure. Everyone has their quirks.

(Annotation: Light explanation, almost a placeholder. The humour prevents contact. On the surface engaged, in depth avoided.)

THERAPIST: I wonder if the checking got worse after the fall-out with your friend.
ELI: (shrugs, laughs lightly): Nah, people argue. It's normal. Not a big deal.

(Annotation: The retreat shows itself. The shrug and laugh deflect weight. I feel the subject closing down, the session staying light but thin.)

THERAPIST: Sometimes things can look small on the outside but still leave a mark inside. Could that be true for you?
ELI: (pause, softer voice): Maybe. I just … don't like the idea he's upset with me.

(Annotation: The minimisation cracks. A flicker of guilt comes through once the mood is gently held. This took several sessions to reach, showing how retreat can loosen with patience.)

Commentary

The transcripts show that Eli and Amira have a psychic retreat position to their OCD. It is not marked by absence of speech or by overt collapse, but by a thinning of emotional presence. What is most striking is the subtlety of the shift. Amira maintains poise, Eli sustains humour, and both appear engaged. Yet in each case, the therapist feels the atmosphere flatten or the conversation skim away from affect. The retreat is revealed less in what is said than in the way it is said, and in the countertransference it evokes.

For the clinician, these moments are often confusing. There is the temptation to praise maturity, to accept minimisation, or to push for disclosure. The retreat calls for something different: patient recognition that compulsions have stepped in as substitutes for feelings. Naming this pattern gently, and noticing the timing of symptoms in relation to emotions, are ways of keeping the channel open without breaking trust.

The commentary section therefore highlights a paradox of the psychic retreat: it often looks like progress because the adolescent is articulate and willing to talk. Yet the very polish of their account may be the sign that feeling has been avoided. Recognising this paradox is key to working clinically with the retreat.

How the Psychic Retreat Appears in the Room

When I first began to notice that obsessive-compulsive symptoms often intensified as a way of working through difficult feelings, I looked for a way to capture this pattern. The idea of the psychic retreat felt closest to what I was seeing. It made intuitive and practical sense to think of this not just as a symptom pattern but as a psychic position in its own right.

Other psychoanalytic writers have described similar dynamics. Betty Joseph (1975) talked about patients who are 'hard to reach', where layers of defence make the therapeutic space feel flat or disconnected. Herbert Rosenfeld (1987) wrote about 'destructive narcissism', where a patient leans into a sense of omnipotence to avoid the vulnerability of dependency. Bion (1959), too, described 'attacks on linking' moments when the usual connections between feelings, thoughts, and events break down because those links are simply too painful to bear. These ideas all resonate, but they didn't quite explain what I was seeing: a particular kind of withdrawal, focused around compulsions, that seemed to act as a last-ditch effort to manage overwhelming emotion, right at the moment when thinking about it became too much

Emotional Fluctuation

Young people in this position often show stretches of genuine emotional availability. They may reflect openly on their rituals when life feels calm. Yet, when conflict or a charged feeling surfaces, the atmosphere changes quickly. The same adolescent who was lively last week arrives this week flat, overly compliant, or oddly light-hearted, even while symptoms have spiked.

What is interesting here is that emotional fluctuation is part and parcel of adolescence, and it is important not to mistake every swing in mood for evidence of a psychic retreat. Some feelings are simply harder to talk about than others. One adolescent may speak freely about sexual feelings but avoid anger altogether; another may be able to explore guilt yet fall silent at the mention of desire. The difference in the psychic retreat is that the fluctuation is not random. It tends to be linked to the moments when something difficult is happening, either externally in relationships or internally in the adolescent's mind. As a clinician, you can find yourself looking forward to a session after a good week, only to feel that the atmosphere has closed down the next. The clue is in the timing: the emotional withdrawal coincides with the return of intrusive thoughts and compulsions, as if ritual has stepped in to take the place of feeling that could not be borne.

Sidestepping of Affect

Adolescents in this position can often give detailed accounts of their week, describe their rituals clearly, and even appear reflective. Yet the telling is curiously flat. Key emotional notes are skipped or smoothed over. An argument at home may be described as 'normal', or a humiliation at school brushed aside with, 'It's fine now.' The narrative holds together but the feeling is missing.

What matters here is not to mistake this for resilience or maturity. Adolescents vary widely in how they talk about emotions, and many will naturally prefer a more cognitive or story-based style. In the psychic retreat, however, the consistent avoidance of affect stands out. The account is not simply factual; it is hollowed of feeling at the very points where feeling would be expected. I often notice myself drawn in by the apparent coherence, only later realising that what has been omitted carries more weight than what was said. The ritual often fills the gap, as if it is holding the unspoken feeling.

What can be exceptionally difficult is that a young person may describe a conflict in such a mature and sophisticated way that I feel pulled to compliment them for thinking so rationally and reasonably. When this happens once, it may be a genuine sign of development. When it happens again and again, across different dilemmas and interpersonal stresses, and every time the responses are cool, logical, and detached from feeling, something else is at work. The repeated smoothness is often the sign. At that point, I begin to suspect I am not just engaging with a thoughtful adolescent but with one who is skilfully sidestepping affect because allowing it in would feel too overwhelming or messy and might activate or intensify their obsessive and compulsive symptoms.

Symptom Escalation after Emotional Triggers

OCD symptoms often surge immediately after a difficult emotional event. Yet, when asked, the adolescent explains the increase in cognitive terms:

'exam stress', 'poor sleep', or 'just random'. The timing feels too exact to ignore, but the link is denied.

Here, I feel the pull of a split. Part of me wants to accept the rational explanation, while another part senses that the compulsions are acting as a smokescreen. The retreat replaces unbearable emotion with ritual detail. What makes this challenging is that the young person may not be fully aware of the feelings that came before the obsessions and compulsions. Some emotions are complex and harder to recognise, such as guilt, disappointment, or envy. Others, like rage or hatred, can feel so dangerous to the adolescent's self-image that they are warded off before they can be thought about. In adolescence, when emotional impulses are already heightened and intensified, these experiences can feel overwhelming.

It is not that the adolescent is deliberately trying to deceive the clinician. More often, it is that they do not want to think about what the symptoms might be linked to. Bion's description of 'attacks on linking' (1959) comes to mind: the severing of the natural connections between event, feeling, and thought. In the psychic retreat, compulsions and intrusive thoughts can serve this function. They attack the possibility of linking because the idea of making the link is itself unbearable. A young person may feel massive envy toward a friend, or rage toward a teacher, or impulses that feel alien to their character. To recognise the feeling and connect it to the event would feel too dangerous, so the connection is cut. In its place, the obsessive and compulsive symptoms intensify, providing both an explanation and a defence.

Polite but Protected

These adolescents are often warm, agreeable, and even insightful. They nod, agree, and may say, 'That makes sense,' or 'I'll try that.' Yet the conversation does not deepen. The defence is polished avoidance.

As therapist, I can find myself colluding with this surface compliance, enjoying the likable manner while knowing the real work has been kept just out of reach. Outside the room, the compulsions carry what was not spoken.

In my experience, these young people often instil hopefulness and optimism at first because they are engaging. They may be willing to describe their obsessions and compulsions in detail, even the more sensitive intrusive thoughts, and they can articulate them in ways that feel thoughtful and meaningful. Some cite psychoeducation they have read or recall strategies they have learnt. They are often adolescents one can connect with quite readily.

The challenge comes when emotion enters the room. At that point, the engagement thins, and the polished avoidance appears. This becomes especially significant when exposure and response prevention is introduced too quickly. On paper, the adolescent may report positive results: they exposed themselves, resisted the compulsion, and 'proved' they could tolerate distress.

Progress looks promising. Yet in practice, those weeks of apparent success often coincide with a period in which conflict, guilt, embarrassment, or vulnerability have been kept at bay. The rituals may reduce, but only because the underlying emotional triggers have not been stirred.

This is why cases of psychic retreat can appear deceptively successful. They may be discharged with encouraging reports, only to return later when the next stage of development forces the avoided feelings back into view. At that point, symptoms escalate sharply, sometimes leaving the clinician puzzled or disheartened that previous gains did not hold. In truth, the work was never false. Talking openly about OCD is valuable. But the deeper avoidance of feeling means the progress was conditional, dependent on whether certain emotions remained out of reach. That conditionality is itself a sign that the adolescent was working from within a psychic retreat.

Rituals as Substitutes for Feelings

Compulsions in this position, whether mental or behavioural, are less about preventing external catastrophe and more about regulating inner states. Mental reviewing, moral checking, ordering, or covert reassurance-seeking all function to sedate emotions that feel unmanageable.

The pattern is often clear when rituals intensify precisely at the point when guilt, envy, or anger surface. What cannot yet be felt is sealed inside the ritual. I often notice myself trying to pull the session back toward the underlying emotion, only to find it has already been diverted into compulsion.

As a clinician, I sometimes feel almost obsessive myself, repeatedly trying to return the focus to emotion. Each time, the adolescent may intellectualise it, explain the external event that caused it, and offer a rational justification for why they felt that way. Yet if I ask whether they can link that emotion to the surge in intrusive thoughts or compulsions, they either draw a blank or retreat further, sometimes changing the subject altogether.

This is significant for the psychic retreat: the compulsions themselves are used as emotion regulation. They become a way to work through feelings that feel too strong to manage directly. Take guilt as an example. Guilt can stir the thought, 'I am bad,' or 'I am not a good person.' This can be unbearable to sit with. Working through it in compulsions temporarily reduces the emotional intensity. Yet, if asked directly, the adolescent may brush it aside with a casual, 'Everyone feels guilty sometimes.' The more useful questions are not whether they feel guilt, but what guilt means to them, what they picture when they feel guilty, and how it feels inside.

There are many ways compulsions regulate emotion, but what marks the psychic retreat is that this function is central. Compared with other positions, emotion regulation through compulsion is the defining feature.

> ### Box 9.1 Recognising the Psychic Retreat Position
>
> - Engagement can be warm and thoughtful when calm, but suddenly flattens when feelings rise.
> - Narratives are coherent but stripped of emotional tone.
> - Rituals spike after conflict, guilt, anger, envy, shame, or even excitement.
> - Polite and agreeable on the surface, but deeper exploration is quietly avoided
> - Compulsions function as substitutes for feelings, not as protection against external catastrophe.

Working Clinically

Working with adolescents in a psychic retreat position requires a stance that honours their capacity for functioning while staying curious about the cost of that functioning. These are not young people who refuse to engage. They engage selectively. The retreat is a way of managing what feels unbearable, and therapy must recognise both its usefulness and its limits.

The task for the therapist is to stay present at the threshold. The adolescent is already in the room, but not always willing to remain when a difficult feeling rises. At times, the work feels full of hope. At other times, the atmosphere flattens and connection slips away. What follows are clinical stances I return to in this position. They are not techniques to apply, but ways of being that help the adolescent test whether closeness can be tolerated without retreat.

Naming the Pattern without Accusation

Adolescents in a psychic retreat often feel that their shifts are invisible. Simply noticing and naming them can be transformative, provided it is done gently. I might say, 'When things are calm you are very present here. When something stirs, it feels as if a part of you steps back,' or, 'There seems to be a version of you that handles everything so well, and another part that pulls away when it feels too much.'

These kinds of comments invite reflection rather than defence. They frame the retreat as a signal rather than a failure. The adolescent begins to see the pattern as meaningful, not shameful.

Naming emotions, and naming what is happening in the room, is part of all therapeutic modalities, but it is particularly pertinent in a psychic retreat position. The challenge is to frame it as a gentle observation, not a criticism. If it is heard as pointing out something the adolescent has 'missed' or been 'blind' to, it risks reinforcing shame.

The art is to keep a curious stance. I might say, 'I noticed that ...,' or, 'It may have slipped your mind but I am just noticing ...,' or, 'Could it be that when you feel this, something else happens?' These comments plant a seed without making a demand. They are not confrontations, but small openings. Even if the adolescent is not yet aware of the feelings being regulated by their compulsions, the therapist can model awareness by stepping back and commenting lightly.

In my experience, this works best when such remarks are integrated throughout sessions rather than delivered as a single intervention. Over time, gentle observations accumulate, and the adolescent begins to notice that their rituals are linked to the ebb and flow of difficult feelings. In a position where avoidance is the default, curiosity itself becomes therapeutic.

Tracking the Function, Not Just the Form

Compulsions in this position often act less as barriers against catastrophe and more as sedatives for intolerable emotion. The task is to shift the focus from what the adolescent does to what the ritual does for them. I might say, 'When you replay the conversation in your head, does it help with guilt, even for a moment?' or, 'It sounds as though lining things up makes the feeling settle inside, not just the desk look tidy.'

This approach prevents the session from getting stuck in the mechanics of compulsion. It reframes the ritual as communication, a sign of emotional overload rather than just a habit to extinguish. It also takes a slightly different angle from the usual focus on what triggered the intrusive thought. Instead, we start with the feeling that follows when the compulsion has been carried out successfully. Many adolescents will describe frustration or even anger if a compulsion is interrupted or done incorrectly. But if the ritual is completed in full, without disruption, what is the feeling then?

Exploring this question allows us to see how compulsions are recruited at the very moments when a feeling is difficult to process or think about. If the compulsion works, it is because it has managed an affect, not simply because it has neutralised a thought. Naming this openly can be a turning point. It helps the young person begin to see their compulsions as serving a purpose, regulating feelings that feel too messy or overwhelming to sit with.

Like the other interventions described here, this way of working has to be interwoven gradually throughout sessions. These are not grand interpretations but micro-interventions, each planting the idea that compulsions can be thought about as affect regulation. Over time, this builds a deeper awareness of what the rituals are really doing, and opens space to begin thinking about the feelings themselves.

Making Micro-contact with Emotion

Young people in retreat are not absent. They are watchful. They are testing whether the clinician can bear what they fear they cannot. The task is not to pull them into emotional exposure but to help them try small doses of contact. I might say, 'It sounded like you almost said something, then stopped. Shall we see what happens if you let it out a little?' Or, 'You mentioned the argument quickly. I wonder if there's a feeling nearby that we could name together, without having to stay there too long.'

This intervention is all about working in the here and now. That is true of therapy generally, but in the psychic retreat the work requires a particular alertness to the smallest shifts: a half-finished sentence, a sudden sigh, clenched fists, a restless movement when a topic comes close to something raw. The role of the therapist is to signal that these shifts are noticed without being too intrusive. In practice, this means letting the young person know that I am aware of what is stirring, even if they are not ready to name it.

Sometimes, I will share a small piece of my own imagined feeling in a neutral, universal situation. For example, I might say, 'When a friend agrees to meet me and then cancels at the last minute, I know it is not their fault, but I still feel frustrated.' This kind of self-disclosure is not about redirecting the focus to me. It is a way of modelling that frustration, disappointment, or guilt are ordinary feelings that can be thought about without collapse. Even a flicker of contact, when tolerated in this way, reduces the need to retreat.

The art is to do this in a manner that feels tentative, light, and safe. If the therapist jumps in too quickly, the adolescent may feel overwhelmed and step further back. If it is done with curiosity and patience, the adolescent begins to discover that small steps toward feeling can be survived, and that the room can hold whatever emerges.

Validating the Function of the Retreat

The psychic retreat has been necessary for survival. To dismantle it too quickly risks confirming that closeness is unsafe. I might say, 'It makes sense that your mind found a safe place to go when it felt too much,' or, 'This pattern has probably protected you at difficult times. We can respect that even as we look at whether it is still needed.'

Validating the defence helps the adolescent feel less ashamed of using it, and paradoxically makes them more willing to test moments of contact. Obsessive-compulsive symptoms themselves can be thought of as compromised formations, attempts to manage experiences that feel too intense to acknowledge directly. The psychic retreat is one such formation. It is a way to survive, just as the claustrum is a way to survive by cutting off, and the paranoid–schizoid position is a way to survive by projecting danger outward.

This framing matters. If we treat the retreat simply as pathology, we miss its protective logic. When we honour it as a survival strategy, we can begin to explore both what it provides and what it costs. The function is usually clear: it shields the adolescent from emotional overwhelm, from guilt that feels unbearable, from anger that might damage others, or from vulnerability that feels too exposing. But the cost is equally important: the retreat blocks growth, prevents emotional connection, and leaves compulsions to carry what cannot be faced.

In practice, the intervention is to name the retreat without using the jargon, to wonder aloud about what it does, and then to invite reflection on what it costs. This has to be done tentatively, in small steps. The adolescent needs to feel that their retreat is respected before they can risk loosening it. Done carefully, this approach helps them see that while the retreat has kept them safe, it cannot be the only strategy for living.

Testing the Edges Gently

Progress in this position is not about abolishing the retreat, but about testing whether it is possible to stay near the edge of it without collapse. I might ask, 'If we stayed with this feeling for just a minute longer, what do you imagine might happen?' or, 'It is as if the feeling is waiting outside the door. Shall we peek together, or keep the door closed today?' These kinds of experiments help the adolescent approach feelings symbolically rather than directly. The aim is proximity, not endurance. Each attempt makes the retreat less absolute and emotional contact more thinkable.

One of the most challenging aspects of therapy, particularly with adolescents, is helping them to sit with feelings that are difficult to bear. The instinct is often to numb or distract. A phone screen, a game, a stream, or a substance can offer immediate escape. This automatic retreat from feeling is part of adolescent life, but in the psychic retreat position it is crystallised into compulsive form. The rituals are called on in the same way a screen might be: as a fast route away from pain.

Once a secure therapeutic relationship has been established, and once it has been recognised that the adolescent's stance toward their OCD fits the psychic retreat, the work becomes helping them to tolerate a little more. The task is to notice a feeling and stay with it, to see what effect it has on the body, and to observe what happens in their behaviour. This does not mean rushing to expression or catharsis. It means helping them test what it feels like to linger, even briefly, at the edge of retreat.

Over time, this can reduce the need for compulsions to serve as full emotional regulators. If a young person can tolerate a flicker of guilt, anger, or envy without retreat, the ritual may no longer need to do all the work. They may still use compulsions, but for shorter periods, or with less urgency, because they have already managed to sit with some of the feeling themselves. In this way, the retreat is not dismantled in one piece, but gradually loosened as the adolescent learns that emotions can be survived in the room.

Reframing Progress in Therapy

Progress in the psychic retreat is subtle and easily missed. It may not show itself in reduced compulsion scores or dramatic shifts in functioning. Instead, it looks like a feeling named instead of deflected, a silence tolerated rather than filled, a retreat noticed before it fully takes hold, a ritual recognised as carrying a feeling, or a young person who left last week returning this week.

Beyond the reduction of obsessive–compulsive symptoms, this position offers the possibility of deeper growth. The retreat is, at its core, a way of managing emotions. When a young person begins to tolerate more of those emotions directly, the compulsions lose some of their urgency. Progress is measured in the ability to sit with a difficult feeling, to endure a silence, to permit emotions that once felt destructive, anger, rage, despair, without believing they will shatter relationships or destroy the self.

These shifts can be more important than symptom reduction alone. If the adolescent learns that when big feelings arrive, they no longer have to retreat into ritual, then the OCD has already loosened. Emotions begin to function as a compass, not as dangers to be avoided. Progress in this position should therefore never be reduced to the absence of symptoms, although that will always remain a welcome indicator. The deeper therapeutic work, and the gains that are most likely to last, come from the ability to recognise one's feelings, tolerate them, and resist the pull to retreat from them.

Guidance for Parents

(*For clinicians to use when communicating with families.*)

When I speak with parents about the psychic retreat, I describe it as a kind of internal safe room. From the outside, their child may look engaged – attending school, brushing their teeth, joining family meals – but inside they have stepped back. They are surviving by retreating from feelings that feel too intense.

Parents are often puzzled because their adolescent appears high functioning. The idea of the retreat helps to name what feels absent without placing blame on the young person.

I might say to families: 'Sometimes when feelings get too strong, young people find a quiet internal place to hide. From the outside they may look fine, but emotionally they are not fully present,' or, 'When the OCD gets louder, it can be a sign that your child has stepped into that safe room. The rituals are not laziness or defiance. They are a way of coping with something that feels too big to face.' And sometimes, 'You do not need to force them out. You just need to let them know the door can stay open, and you are there when they step back out.'

At the same time, I am mindful that not all parents will respond to metaphors like safe rooms or islands of the mind. Some parents need the explanation in more grounded, concrete terms. With them, I emphasise that OCD symptoms often flare up when something difficult is happening emotionally. Instead of naming, tolerating, or processing the difficulty, whether it is a feeling, a reaction, or a situation, the young person turns to ritual. I explain that things may seem fine for weeks, then symptoms surge again. This is usually the point at which new feelings have been stirred.

Classic examples include the ups and downs of early relationships. A new romance may feel exciting until expectations deepen, jealousy arises, or a breakup occurs. Rivalry with peers, humiliation in social settings, or disappointment at home can all trigger the same process. When these feelings surface and feel unmanageable, OCD symptoms often intensify.

The task for parents is not to interrogate or force disclosure, but to hold a stance of curiosity. I encourage them to think: 'If the OCD is worse, what feelings might have come up for my child?' Naming this to themselves, or gently opening a space for their child to speak if they wish, is often enough. Even if the adolescent does not want to talk, the parental stance of tolerance and presence communicates safety.

When parents are more psychologically minded, I may use the metaphorical language of rooms, islands, or internal places of retreat. When they are less so, I stick with the simple truth: something has felt too much, and the OCD has stepped in to help the adolescent cope. Both ways are true to the concept of the psychic retreat. The choice is about meeting parents where they are and giving them language that makes sense in their world.

Summary and Clinical Take Home

The psychic retreat is not a fortress. It is a sanctuary assembled when needed, dismantled when calm returns, and held together by rituals, avoidance, and careful self-presentation. On the surface, it looks like coping. Beneath the surface, it is a conditional withdrawal, where intrusive thoughts and compulsions step forward to take the place of feelings that feel too raw or risky to face.

This position is easily missed in systems that value attendance, compliance, and performance. These adolescents can look fine. They arrive on time, they nod, they complete tasks, and they may even reflect thoughtfully. Yet their emotional presence is conditional. They are in the room until a feeling approaches, then they step back.

For the therapist, this can be both promising and elusive. One moment there is warmth and genuine engagement. The next, the atmosphere flattens and the adolescent slips away behind a polite exterior. The sense of loss is mirrored in the countertransference. I notice in myself a quiet disappointment, as if something precious has been withdrawn. This mirroring is not incidental. It is part of the structure of the retreat.

The work is not to drag the adolescent out or to dismantle the retreat by force. It is to remain steady at the threshold. The smallest steps matter: a feeling named rather than avoided, a silence tolerated rather than filled, a ritual recognised for what it is doing. These are not minor shifts. They are the footholds on which deeper work rests.

When the adolescent can test staying in contact a little longer without collapse, the retreat begins to loosen. With time and safety, this often opens the way toward the depressive position, where guilt and ambivalence can finally be acknowledged and worked with directly. The retreat is therefore not the end of development but a transitional defence, one that points toward the possibility of mourning, repair, and more enduring connection.

Box 9.2 ERP and the Psychic Retreat: When to Pause and When to Proceed

- Exposure and response prevention (ERP) may appear possible: the adolescent is articulate, engaged, and can describe their compulsions clearly.
- Apparent 'success' with early ERP may be misleading, as it often coincides with calm periods when difficult feelings are absent.
- Readiness is best judged after an emotional trigger: does the adolescent stay present, or do they withdraw into ritual?
- If rituals spike immediately after conflict, guilt, or shame, ERP should be delayed until these links can be thought about.
- Short exposures can be used as gentle tests, but monitor whether they bypass feeling (done smoothly, but without depth).
- True readiness emerges when the adolescent can tolerate discussion of the feelings beneath symptoms, even briefly.
- Without this, ERP risks becoming another layer of polished avoidance – reported as progress but fragile and reversible.

Box 9.3 Clinician's Guidance to Parents

- The young person may seem articulate and fine on the surface, but symptoms often flare when difficult feelings (guilt, shame, anger, envy) are stirred.
- Do not assume the OCD has gone just because things look calmer – the retreat is temporary, not a cure.
- Avoid pressing for emotional disclosure; over-probing can trigger withdrawal.
- Keep family communication steady and low in intensity. Small, ordinary contact is more useful than heavy questioning.
- Notice and praise balanced effort, not only symptom reduction.
- Understand that rituals here often serve to regulate feelings, not to prevent catastrophe – this helps you frame them without blame.
- Offer reassurance sparingly: what helps most is calm presence and acceptance, not repeated 'Are you okay?' checks.

References

Bion, W. R. (1959). Attacks on linking. *International Journal of Psycho-Analysis*, 40, 308–315.

Joseph, B. (1975). The patient who is difficult to reach. In P. L. Giovacchini (Ed.), *Tactics and techniques in psychoanalytic therapy*, Volume 2: Countertransference (pp. 109–121). Lanham, MD: Jason Aronson.

Rosenfeld, H. (1987). *Impasse and interpretation: Therapeutic and anti-therapeutic factors in the psychoanalytic treatment of psychotic, borderline and neurotic patients.* London and New York: Routledge.

Steiner, J. (1993). *Psychic retreats: Pathological organizations in psychotic, neurotic and borderline patients.* London and New York: Routledge.

Chapter 10

The Paranoid–Schizoid Position in OCD

It is a hot day in the consulting room. Two fans are blowing to circulate the air. After lunch, I feel the pull of a midday slump, yet the 16-year-old girl in front of me seems oblivious to the temperature. She speaks in an anxious flurry. 'I was so close to touching something I was terrified. I genuinely thought I was going to drop dead.'

She goes on to describe contaminated objects and her fear that others might 'make her' get ill or stop her from completing her rituals. Despite my post-lunch crash, my mind is suddenly alert. I can feel the anxiety in the room as if there really is a threat outside, as if she could genuinely be harmed by not touching a table an even number of times.

This is the atmosphere of the paranoid–schizoid position.

Conceptual Overview: Understanding the Paranoid–Schizoid Position

Melanie Klein, writing in 1946, described it as one of the mind's earliest ways of organising experience in infancy. The world is felt in stark contrasts: good or bad, safe or unsafe, pure or contaminated. Experience is divided into opposites with little space for ambiguity, a process known as 'splitting' described in Chapter 3 as one of infancy's earliest defensive mechanisms. In those early months, splitting allows the mind to cope with overwhelming feelings by keeping love and hate, comfort and fear, firmly apart.

This way of perceiving the world is not confined to infancy. It is something all of us revert to when under strain. In moments of stress or anxiety we may fall into black-and-white thinking, lose our capacity to hold nuance, and feel as though danger is absolute. In that sense, the paranoid–schizoid way of organising experience is a universal human response.

What distinguishes the adolescents I describe here is not that they occasionally split, but that this state of mind becomes the organising framework for their obsessive-compulsive disorder (OCD). It solidifies into a psychic position. Intrusive thoughts are not fleeting intrusions; they are treated as

DOI: 10.4324/9781003729716-10

literal proofs of danger, corruption, or guilt. Compulsions then follow as urgent safety devices, pressed into service to hold the danger at bay.

In OCD, the paranoid–schizoid position therefore moves beyond an ordinary stress reaction. It becomes a fixed way of living in the world, where threat feels constant and catastrophic, and where rituals must be enacted to preserve safety. This is what makes the position so compelling in the consulting room and so exhausting for the young person who inhabits it.

Time must be invested in containing and symbolising the external threat and the terror it produces. Only when a sense of safety can be established within the therapeutic frame does exposure and response prevention (ERP) become possible. Introduced too early, it risks collapse or reinforcement of the defence. Introduced at the right moment, once safety is felt and the fear has been held symbolically, ERP may carry a far higher chance of success.

The following clinical examples illustrate how the paranoid–schizoid position can appear in practice. What stands out is not just the content of the intrusive thoughts, but the atmosphere they generate in the room. The fear is carried as if it were literal fact, and the compulsion is enacted as the only possible safeguard. As a therapist, I find myself drawn into the urgency, feeling the same pressure to reassure, to argue, or to prove safety that the young person is already trapped in. These cases show how easily we can be recruited into the logic of the defence, and how much work is required to hold the terror without collusion.

Clinical Examples of the Paranoid–Schizoid Position in OCD

Liam

Liam, a 13-year-old boy, was referred after his parents noticed he avoided the bathroom and would only shower late at night. In our first sessions, he spoke hesitantly but clearly about intrusive thoughts of sin and evil. These thoughts clung to anything involving nudity or bodily fluids, and he described them as proof that something inside him was corrupt.

His family's religious background gave him some language for these fears, but Liam's conviction went far beyond doctrine. He was certain that, if he did not wash in a precise way, something bad would happen. When I tentatively suggested that thoughts might not equal actions, he replied, 'That sounds like something people say when they're lying to you.'

My own countertransference was immediate: I felt pulled into the role of defender, almost arguing on behalf of his innocence. Each time I tried to reassure, his resistance hardened. This is the paranoid–schizoid position at its clearest. The danger is lived as literal, not hypothetical, and any attempt to soften it is met with suspicion. Unlike the claustrum, where the feared danger often remains vague, Liam could describe in detail what would happen if he 'got it wrong'.

Progress only began when I shifted from reassurance to curiosity. Together, we explored how anger toward his brother felt unbearable, and how the thought of being 'bad' was displaced into rituals of cleansing. ERP was only possible once Liam felt I could bear his certainty without rushing to undo it. The turning point was not washing less, but allowing himself to admit that he sometimes hated his brother – and discovering that did not make him evil, just human.

Nina

Nina, a 15-year-old girl, came with relentless checking rituals. She feared she had left the oven on, forgotten to lock the door, or endangered her pet. She would text her parents repeatedly for reassurance or retrace her steps to check appliances.

In session she was warm and talkative, sometimes even humorous, but beneath it all there was a constant sense of dread. She described a gnawing conviction that something terrible was about to happen and that she would be to blame. When I asked how she knew it was real, she said, 'Because the feeling means it's real.'

This became especially clear after emotional events. Following a fight with a friend, her checking surged: 30 times at the light switch, repeated messages to her parents. When I asked about the argument, she shrugged, 'I don't care.' Then, almost in the same breath, she asked whether I had checked the office kettle. The emotional link was obvious, though she could not name it directly.

Sitting with Nina, I often felt pulled into her vigilance – double-checking my own words, as though one slip might cause the catastrophe she dreaded. It was a mirror of her inner world: tense, watchful, certain that danger was imminent.

Unlike the psychic retreat, where emotional contact is lost when things get too raw, Nina remained engaged, but her engagement was ruled by dread. Therapy turned toward connecting the spikes in her compulsions with moments of shame, guilt, or conflict. Progress was not a dramatic reduction in checking, but Nina beginning to see that her rituals were less about switches and ovens, and more about unbearable feelings she could not yet tolerate.

Clinical Transcripts

Liam (Paranoid–Schizoid Position)

Context: Liam has been describing his intrusive fears about sin and evil, alongside compulsive washing rituals. The therapist is exploring how literal these fears feel, and how reassurance is received.

THERAPIST: You've told me you sometimes have thoughts you describe as 'bad'. Can you say more about what makes them bad?

LIAM: (hesitant): They just … come. About hurting people. About sex. I know they mean I'm evil.

(Annotation: His words are heavy with conviction. There is no sense of 'maybe' here. The thought is experienced as a direct truth about who he is.)

THERAPIST: You sound very certain. What do you imagine would happen if you didn't try to wash those thoughts away?

LIAM: (quickly): Something bad will happen. I'll be punished. I'll go to hell.

(Annotation: Unlike the claustrum, where the feared outcome is often vague or absent, Liam can describe the consequence with precision. His danger is externalised and moral, experienced as literal fact.)

THERAPIST: Some people find it helps to think of thoughts as just thoughts, not as proof of who they are.

LIAM: (interrupts): That's what people say when they're lying to you.

(Annotation: His mistrust lands sharply. In me it stirs an urge to defend him, to prove his innocence. I notice how easily I get drawn into reassurance – and how futile it feels.)

THERAPIST: It sounds hard to believe me when I say the thought isn't proof you're bad.

LIAM: (looks down): I can't take the risk. What if it's true?

(Annotation: Here the paranoid–schizoid position shows its grip. There is no space for ambivalence – either he is good or he is evil. The compulsion becomes the only way to push away that unbearable uncertainty.)

THERAPIST: Maybe part of what the washing does is give you a break from that fear. But perhaps it also keeps you from finding out that the thought doesn't make you bad.

(Annotation: I resist the pull to reassure, instead naming the function of the ritual gently. The work is to stay beside his certainty without colluding with it.)

Nina (Paranoid–Schizoid Position)

Context: Nina's compulsions have intensified after a falling-out with a close friend. She insists the two are unrelated. The therapist suspects her checking rituals are a defence against unbearable guilt and self-blame.

THERAPIST: You mentioned you've been checking your bedroom light switch more often this week – maybe 20 times before bed?
NINA: (quickly): Yeah. I just couldn't remember if I turned it off. I was tired.

(Annotation: Her answer is brisk, almost rehearsed. The speed itself feels defensive, as though she is trying to head off further exploration before I can make the connection.)

THERAPIST: Being tired makes sense. But usually when you're tired, you let it go. Something feels different this week.
NINA: (shrugs): I don't know. Maybe I'm just being extra careful.

(Annotation: The shrug is familiar here – not avoidance in the claustral sense, but a protective half-answer. She wants to appear engaged while keeping me away from what really hurts.)

THERAPIST: Carefulness seems to help you feel a bit more in control. Maybe because something inside didn't feel in control?
NINA: (avoids eye contact): I guess I was annoyed at Alice. She said I was being dramatic. I wasn't mad, just ... embarrassed.

(Annotation: This is the shift. Her gaze drops and the tone softens. The compulsions are not about switches or light bulbs – they are about humiliation, anger, and the terror of being judged 'too much'.)

THERAPIST: Sometimes when we feel dismissed or embarrassed, it's easier to focus on what we can control – like a switch – than to sit with that sting.
NINA: (quietly): It felt like she hated me.

(Annotation: Here the paranoid–schizoid position comes into view: the friend is no longer someone she loves and fights with – she has flipped into enemy. Ambivalence collapses into certainty.)

THERAPIST: That's a painful feeling to carry alone. No wonder your OCD got louder – it may have been trying to distract you from that hurt.

(Annotation: I deliberately stay close to the feeling, naming the link without pressing too hard. The aim is not to prise her out of the defence, but to show that the emotion can be held in the room without catastrophe.)

Commentary

The transcripts show how, in the paranoid–schizoid position, intrusive thoughts are lived not as possibilities but as literal truths. Liam's washing rituals are bound to a moral conviction that he is evil, while Nina's checking spirals from shame and humiliation into catastrophic danger. What is striking is not only the content of their fears, but the certainty with which they are carried. There is no space for ambivalence: either they are safe or doomed, innocent or corrupt, loved or hated.

For the clinician, the countertransference is equally telling. With Liam, I felt the pull to reassure, to defend him against his own verdict of evil. With Nina, I found myself double-checking my words, scanning the session for mistakes in the same way she scanned her world for danger. These responses are not incidental. They mirror the position itself, an atmosphere of vigilance, dread, and pressure to act.

The temptation in these moments is to argue, to soften, or to supply certainty. Yet doing so risks strengthening the cycle. The work instead lies in staying beside the fear without collusion, allowing the ritual to be seen as a defence rather than as proof. Both Liam and Nina illustrate how OCD in this position is less about the specific obsession and more about the collapse of ambivalence, the urgent need to turn 'maybe' into certainty, and the way compulsions are used as safety devices against unbearable feeling.

How the Paranoid–Schizoid Position Appears in the Room

Based on repeated clinical observation, I have identified several indicators that suggest a young person's OCD may be organised through the paranoid–schizoid position. Unlike the claustrum, where withdrawal is global and consistent, or the psychic retreat, where engagement is conditional, the paranoid–schizoid position is marked by vigilance and dread. The adolescent remains engaged, but the contact is charged with urgency. Fear is experienced as literal fact, and compulsions are carried out as safety devices to prevent catastrophe. At times, these young people can even articulate that they know, logically, that their fear is irrational. In this way, the literalness of the fear cannot be dissolved through rational debate alone.

What follows are the hallmarks I have found most useful in recognising when OCD is functioning through a paranoid–schizoid organisation of mind. They do not appear in every case, nor do they form a checklist. They are recurring features in the room, patterns of thought, feeling, and atmosphere, that help us understand when we are working within this position.

Black-and-White Moral Thinking

All of us, under pressure, can fall into black-and-white thinking. It is a universal human response: the mind reduces complexity by dividing the world into good and bad, safe and unsafe. What distinguishes the paranoid–schizoid position in adolescents with OCD is that this splitting becomes the main way of organising intrusive thoughts.

The adolescent voices their fears in stark, moralistic terms. They may say, 'If I thought it, it must be true,' or, 'Good people do not think things like that.' These are not tentative worries but convictions. They shape both the meaning of the intrusive thought and the necessity of the ritual.

There is also an intensity behind this way of thinking. It is a fear-based response. An adolescent who struggles with ambivalence in other positions may simply be unable to think about the space in between, but in the paranoid–schizoid position the refusal of ambivalence is charged with urgency. The feeling is persecutory: 'If I do not act, something terrible will happen.' The splitting carries the texture of dread rather than simple avoidance. In every adolescent I have worked with in this position, the intolerance of ambivalence has been joined by this heightened sense of threat.

Unlike the claustrum, where the feared outcome is vague or absent, here the conviction is sharp and concrete. The splitting of good and bad is not simply an idea but saturates the atmosphere of the room, shaping how both adolescent and clinician think and feel.

Fear Experienced as Literal

What is perhaps most apparent about this position is the presence of a named external threat. Compared with the claustrum, where the feared danger is either absent or only vaguely described, in the paranoid–schizoid position the danger can be pinpointed with striking precision. The adolescent may not share all the details in the first few sessions, while trust is still being established, but when they do it is concrete and specific. Objects, situations, or even particular people can be identified as dangerous in ways that leave little ambiguity.

In this position, fear is not entertained as a possibility, it is lived as fact. The intrusive thought is not 'just a thought' but proof of catastrophe. 'What if I harm my mum?' is not a hypothetical worry, it is felt as imminent reality unless the compulsion is performed.

Many adolescents even acknowledge the irrationality: 'I know it is stupid, I know it is not going to happen, but …' The but marks the split between knowing and feeling. Rationally, they can argue against the fear, but emotionally, the conviction remains untouched. At times, they can even state, with striking clarity, that logically they know the catastrophe will not occur. They may say, 'I know I will not die if I do not wash,' or, 'I know the house will not burn down if I only check once.' Yet the felt sense outweighs logic. The body insists on catastrophe even when the mind can acknowledge otherwise.

This is probably one of the most frustrating aspects for parents and primary caregivers. The young person can say how stupid their ideas are, how unlikely and unrealistic, and yet they keep doing them. The natural instinct of parents is to ask, "If you know it is not real, why do you keep doing it?" They may begin to suspect the adolescent is doing it on purpose, or that their

OCD is not as serious as it appears. This often leads to more challenges, more pressure, or repeated statements like, 'You know it's not real, so just stop.' While often well meant, these comments can be detrimental. They increase shame and leave the young person feeling both misunderstood and trapped.

What I have found most helpful in the consulting room is to name the discrepancy directly. I often say something like, 'I hear you say you know it will not happen, and at the same time it still feels as if it will.' Naming the gap between the logical understanding and the felt conviction validates the experience. It shows the young person they are not fraudulent, that their insight and their fear can co-exist, and that this very split is what makes the position so exhausting.

What gives the position its particular texture is the persecutory edge. The adolescent is not simply unable to tolerate ambivalence, as may be the case in other positions. Here, the refusal of ambivalence is driven by urgency and dread. The conviction is not only strong, it is compelling, as if the adolescent were already standing at the edge of disaster.

When Rituals Become Safety Devices

Once the threat has been named and carried as fact, compulsions take on the role of safety devices. In the paranoid–schizoid position, the ritual is not just a way of soothing tension or restoring inner balance, it is lived as the only thing standing between the adolescent and catastrophe.

Checking, confessing, washing, or mental reviewing are carried out with the conviction that if the ritual is not completed something bad will happen. The logic is literal: 'If I do not touch the table four times, my dad will die.' 'If I do not repeat the prayer word-for-word, I will be punished.' The compulsion functions as a shield against real-world danger, not just as a habit or superstition.

This is where the difference between positions becomes clear. In the claustrum, rituals aim to restore a sense of rightness inside the self. In the psychic retreat, rituals flare as a way of pulling back from unbearable emotional intensity. In the paranoid–schizoid position, the danger is felt to be external and imminent, and the ritual is deployed as defence.

For the clinician, the intensity of this conviction is often felt in the countertransference. Sessions can carry a sense of being recruited into the urgency of the ritual. I find myself almost believing that, if the behaviour is not performed, something terrible really will happen. It is in those moments that the paranoid–schizoid organisation of mind shows its power.

Never Switching Off

The tragedy of this position is that even when the external environment is calm, the adolescent cannot relax. Even when there are no obvious threats, no dirty door handles or crowded corridors, they are still anticipating the next contamination or the next danger. Many young people have said to me, 'I can never switch off.'

I remember once commenting that it was interesting that their OCD seemed to rest when they were in a safe place, away from school. They quickly corrected me: 'Even though I am not at school and there are no grubby doors or corridors to touch, I am still thinking about the next corridor, the next classroom, the next situation. I am already planning how I will avoid it.' In this way, the vigilance never pauses. Their minds are locked in a state of hyper-alertness, preparing for threats that have not yet arrived.

The cognitive impact of this constant readiness is immense. It is as if survival depends on anticipating danger at all times. I recall one girl for whom almost everything in her life became a threat. She had only one room at home that felt safe. Everywhere else – the corridor, the landing, the garden, the community – carried the possibility of danger, contamination, or catastrophe if she did not perform a ritual to undo the thought. I remember feeling exhausted just listening to her. The sheer intensity of her vigilance was painful to witness, and it gave me only a glimpse of what it must be like to live inside it all the time.

Box 10.1 Recognising the Paranoid–Schizoid Position

- Rigid good–bad thinking. The adolescent organises the world into absolutes: clean or contaminated, safe or dangerous, pure or sinful, with little tolerance for grey areas.
- Externalised danger. Feelings of guilt, anger, or desire are projected outward and experienced as external threats that must be neutralised through ritual or checking.
- High anxiety and vigilance. The room feels charged. The young person watches closely for reassurance or confirmation, and the therapist often feels pulled to soothe or prove safety.
- Compulsions as protection. Rituals serve as defensive acts to ward off internal chaos, not simply to reduce anxiety; they function as moral or physical safeguards against imagined catastrophe.
- Resistance to symbolic reflection. Attempts to explore meaning are met with literal answers or confusion. Thoughts are treated as facts, not representations, and interpretation may feel intrusive or unsafe.

Working Clinically

Sitting with adolescents in the paranoid–schizoid position is both compelling and exhausting. The threat is named, the fear is lived as fact, and the rituals are performed with a sense of life-or-death necessity. The atmosphere in the room can leave the therapist feeling pressed to deliver certainty, to reassure, or to argue with the logic of the fear. Yet each of those responses risks reinforcing the defence. The task is not to prove safety, but to contain the fear long enough for it to be thought about.

In this section, I describe the therapeutic comments I have found most useful when working in this position. They are not techniques to be applied rigidly but stances that help maintain contact without collusion. Each one addresses a specific clinical challenge: the literalness of the fear, the collapse between thought and action, the function of compulsions, the hunger for certainty, and the emotional undercurrents that so often lie beneath the symptoms.

Respect the Literalness Before Moving to the Symbolic

In the paranoid–schizoid position, intrusive thoughts are not experienced as possibilities but as facts. 'If I thought it, it means it will happen.' 'If I do not carry out the ritual, someone will be harmed.' The natural clinical instinct is to challenge this logic quickly: to reassure, to explain probability, or to remind the young person that thoughts are not the same as actions. Yet, in this position such moves often backfire. The adolescent hears them as dismissive or untrustworthy.

I have found it more effective to begin by respecting the literal quality of the fear. To sit alongside it as it is lived, rather than rushing to dismantle it. Sometimes that means saying something like, 'That sounds terrifying. Carrying that responsibility must feel very heavy.' When the conviction is taken seriously in this way, space slowly opens for symbolic thinking. The fear can start to be considered not only as an external threat, but as something that may also carry meaning about inner states.

The timing of this shift is crucial. Push too soon, and the adolescent doubles down on the literal threat. Move slowly, and the possibility of symbolisation begins to emerge. I often notice in myself the pull to soften their fear, to reassure them into calm. When I resist that urge and allow the fear to be felt in the room, it creates the conditions for the adolescent to begin translating the literal into the symbolic themselves.

This differs from work in the claustrum, where the task is to enliven a sealed-off interior, or in the psychic retreat, where the aim is to stay present at the threshold of withdrawal. In the paranoid–schizoid position, the emotional life is already alive but saturated with catastrophe. The clinical task is not to animate or to hold back, but to stay steady beside the literalness of the fear until it becomes thinkable.

Interrupt the Collapse Between Thought and Action

In the paranoid–schizoid position, thoughts are not experienced as ideas but as imminent actions. 'If I imagined it, it means I want to do it.' 'If the picture came into my head, then it will happen.' The space between thinking and doing collapses, and the adolescent feels compelled to act as though the thought itself were already dangerous.

Clinically, this creates enormous pressure in the room. I often feel an urge to rush in with reassurance – 'Of course you are not going to stab your friend' – or to argue logically against the fusion of thought and action. Yet these responses rarely help. They only reinforce the adolescent's belief that thoughts and deeds are fused, because, if I need to deny it so quickly, then perhaps it really could be true.

Instead, the task is to hold the space open between thought and action. I sometimes say, 'So the thought came. But having the thought is not the same as carrying it out. Can we sit together in that space between the two?' By slowing the moment down, the young person can begin to discover that thoughts can be tolerated without being obeyed.

This differs from the claustrum, where the problem is not the collapse between thought and action but the deadening of thought altogether. In the paranoid–schizoid position, the opposite is true: thought is brimming with meaning, too much meaning, and the urgency is to act before catastrophe strikes. Therapy here is about gently stretching the space between inner event and outer action so that reflection and ambivalence can begin to find room.

Reframe Compulsions as Messages Rather Than Mistakes

Adolescents in the paranoid–schizoid position often see their compulsions as evidence that something is wrong with them. Families and services sometimes reinforce this view, treating the behaviours only as problems to be stopped. When compulsions are seen only as mistakes, the adolescent feels both defective and misunderstood.

In therapy, I have found it helpful to frame compulsions differently: as messages about what cannot yet be spoken. A washing ritual may be a displaced way of managing 'dirty' or shameful feelings. Repeated checking may be a way of holding unbearable responsibility. Confessing may be an attempt to undo guilt or self-blame. The behaviour is not random. It is carrying something that has not yet found words.

I sometimes say to a young person, 'Your OCD is trying to tell us something. Let's see if we can listen to it together.' This shift does not excuse the compulsions, but it allows them to be taken seriously as communication. Instead of trying to extinguish the behaviour straight away, we ask what it might be saying.

The countertransference here is important. I often notice my own pull to tidy things up, to make the ritual go away so the session feels ordered again. But when I resist that impulse, I can begin to hear the compulsion as a message. The very detail that feels repetitive or frustrating may be the closest we can get, in that moment, to the feeling the adolescent cannot yet name.

This contrasts with the claustrum, where rituals are often used to sustain a sealed-off inner 'rightness', and with the psychic retreat, where they act as sedatives against emotional overwhelm. In the paranoid–schizoid position, the compulsion functions as an active defence, a coded communication that tells us something about the danger the adolescent feels compelled to ward off.

Work With the Craving for Certainty

Few things are more striking in the paranoid–schizoid position than the adolescent's hunger for certainty. They want guarantees: that harm will not occur, that their thoughts are not dangerous, that they themselves are not bad. When certainty is withheld, panic rises. When it is given, it provides only brief relief before the cycle repeats.

The therapeutic challenge is to meet this craving without colluding with it or humiliating the part that longs for it. Dismissing the need for certainty – 'No one can ever be 100 per cent sure' – may be factually true, but it risks shaming the adolescent. It tells them that what feels like survival is 'just irrational'. On the other hand, offering endless reassurance strengthens the loop.

I have found it most useful to name the craving itself with compassion: 'I can hear how badly you want to be sure. It makes sense you would look for that. At the same time, I wonder if certainty might be something OCD keeps tricking you into chasing, without ever letting you rest.' In this way, the longing is recognised rather than mocked, and the pressure to resolve it is gently loosened rather than indulged.

In my own countertransference, I often feel the temptation to provide certainty just to relieve the tension. Saying, "You will be fine," or, "That will not happen" feels like the quickest way to calm the room. But when I resist that urge and stay with the craving itself, the adolescent begins to discover that the need for certainty can be noticed and thought about, even without immediate resolution.

This position differs from what we see in the claustrum, where certainty feels rigid but muted, sealed away behind flatness. In the paranoid–schizoid position, the demand for certainty is insistent and pressing. Our task is not to strip it away, but to help the young person test the possibility that 'maybe' can be tolerated, and that absolute safety is not the only way to survive.

Stay Curious About the Emotional Undercurrents

Intrusive thoughts in the paranoid–schizoid position rarely arise in isolation. They are often stirred by emotional experiences that feel too dangerous to face directly – anger, guilt, jealousy, shame, or desire. These feelings are projected outward and reappear as external threats. The adolescent may not say, 'I am furious with my friend,' but instead become convinced, 'If I don't check the light switch 30 times, she will die.'

For the clinician, the task is to keep one eye on these possible emotional currents, without rushing to interpret them too soon. A sudden spike in handwashing may follow a moment of humiliation. A burst of checking may echo the guilt of an argument. These links are rarely made explicitly by the adolescent, but they often surface indirectly, in the timing and intensity of compulsions.

Sometimes, I find myself tempted to take the obsession or compulsion at face value, treating the behaviour as the whole story. When I pause and ask, 'I notice your checking got worse after that fight with Alice. Do you think the two might be connected?' the picture begins to shift. Even if the adolescent denies it at first, the seed is planted that the fear might be carrying more than it shows.

This position requires tolerance of uncertainty on the part of the therapist. The links are not always clear, and not every ritual hides an obvious emotional trigger. The point is not to unmask a hidden meaning straight away, but to hold a posture of curiosity. By modelling that even frightening feelings can be approached thoughtfully, we create a bridge for the adolescent to begin considering that their OCD may be carrying emotional truths rather than only external threats.

This distinguishes the paranoid–schizoid position from the other positions. In the claustrum, the feelings are sealed away and inaccessible. In the psychic retreat, emotions are acknowledged but then quickly fled from. In the paranoid–schizoid position, the feelings are vivid but displaced into threat. Our curiosity keeps alive the possibility that these feelings can be thought about, not only defended against.

Holding the Work Together

Working with adolescents in the paranoid–schizoid position is demanding. The fears are vivid, the rituals urgent, and the pressure in the room to reassure or provide certainty can be overwhelming. What helps is remembering that these young people are not exaggerating or being dramatic. They are describing their reality as it is lived. Our task is to contain that reality without being swallowed by it, and to open small spaces where reflection and ambivalence can re-enter.

Progress is rarely dramatic. It is often measured in moments when the literal is respected long enough for symbolic meaning to be glimpsed, or when the space between thought and action is held open for a little longer than before. Each of these moments matters. They build the foundations for more enduring change.

Parents, too, need support to understand this position. For them, the adolescent's fears can seem both irrational and frustrating, particularly when the young person admits the fear is "stupid" but continues to act on it anyway. Helping parents see that the behaviour is not wilful but defensive, and that their task is containment rather than correction, is often crucial.

Guidance for Parents

(For clinicians to use when communicating with families.)

When I speak with parents about the paranoid–schizoid position, I try to describe it in everyday terms. I might say:

> When your child is caught in this position, everything feels danger-ous. Not metaphorically, but literally. A stray thought or one missed ritual can feel like it will cause catastrophe. This is why you see them repeat checks or washing even when they tell you they 'know' it is irrational.

Parents are often puzzled – and frustrated – by the contradiction. They hear their child admit, 'I know this is silly, I know it won't happen,' yet watch them carry out the ritual anyway. A natural response is to ask, 'If you know that, why are you still doing it?' or to demand that they stop. While understandable, these responses can heighten the young person's fear and shame. What looks like defiance is actually defence.

I often encourage parents to think of the rituals not as wilful habits but as safety devices. For the adolescent, they are experienced as the only thing preventing disaster. Arguing with the logic rarely helps, because the fear is lived as fact. Instead, what helps most is to contain the fear without feeding it.

I suggest some simple principles:

- Validate the feeling, not the fear. For example: 'I can see that feels terrifying' rather than 'That won't happen.'
- Model calm uncertainty. A phrase like, 'I don't know 100 per cent, but I trust we can handle it' acknowledges the worry without providing endless reassurance.
- Avoid debating the logic. Remind parents that the danger is emotional, not rational. Logical arguments alone cannot loosen it.
- Stay close. Presence itself is protective. Parents do not need the perfect words, but their calm and steady availability often matters most.

Clinicians can reassure parents that this is not their failure, nor is it their role to make the fear vanish. Their task is to remain a secure presence, even when the fear makes no sense. In this way, the family helps contain what feels uncontainable, and the adolescent begins to discover that catastrophe can be faced without certainty and without retreating fully into ritual.

Summary and Clinical Take Home

The paranoid–schizoid position in OCD is marked not by absence, but by urgency. The young person is not sealed away, as in the claustrum, nor dipping in and out of presence, as in the psychic retreat. They are vividly present, but their world is saturated with threat. Intrusive thoughts are carried as literal dangers, rituals are pressed into service as safety devices, and the atmosphere in the room is charged with vigilance.

For the clinician, this position is both compelling and exhausting. One feels the pressure to reassure, to deliver certainty, to rescue the adolescent from their dread. Yet it is precisely these impulses that risk colluding with the defence. The work instead is to contain the fear long enough for it to become thinkable: to respect the literal without being trapped in it, to hold the space between thought and action, to reframe compulsions as meaningful signals, and to stay curious about the emotional undercurrents that so often lie beneath the symptom.

Progress in this position is rarely dramatic. It may look like the adolescent tolerating a moment of uncertainty without ritual, or naming a feeling rather than projecting it outward. Each small step is significant, for it begins to soften the splitting and projection that dominate this position. Over time, with safety and consistency, the paranoid–schizoid position can loosen, making space for more complex states of mind.

This is where therapy often begins to touch the depressive position. Here guilt, ambivalence, and loss can be acknowledged and borne, rather than projected outward or defended against with rituals. The shift is not immediate, nor is it ever complete, but it marks a movement toward a mind that can hold contradiction and survive it.

For adolescents caught in the paranoid–schizoid position, survival has meant constant vigilance. Therapy offers them something different: the possibility of resting, even briefly, in a room where catastrophe does not strike simply because it was imagined.

Box 10.2 ERP and the Paranoid-Schizoid: When to Pause and When to Proceed

- Proceed when safety is established. ERP can be effective once trust and containment are in place. The adolescent must feel the therapist can hold the fear without dismissing it.
- Pause if the fear feels literal. When the young person insists that harm will happen rather than might happen, exposure risks reinforcing persecutory anxiety rather than reducing it.
- Proceed with symbolic scaffolding. Begin only after linking the feared situation to its emotional meaning, so the exposure is experienced as exploration, not punishment.

- Pause when reassurance becomes ritualised. If the therapist feels repeatedly drawn to prove safety or offer logic, the work has slipped into collusion with the obsessional system.
- Proceed gradually, with shared curiosity. Small, co-created experiments ('Let's see what happens') foster agency and allow symbolic thinking to re-emerge.
- Pause if contact breaks down. When the therapeutic relationship feels frozen, hostile, or flooded with mistrust, containment must be re-established before any further exposure work.

Box 10.3 Clinician's Guidance to Parents

- Avoid arguing with the logic of the fear. Trying to reason or reassure often strengthens the anxiety. Focus instead on staying calm and present when the fear arises.
- Keep reassurance to a minimum. Repeated reassurance may temporarily soothe but it feeds the cycle. Gentle acknowledgment of distress ('I can see that feels very real for you') is more helpful.
- Maintain emotional steadiness. The young person may shift quickly between trust and suspicion. Parents' consistency helps restore a sense of safety and predictability.
- Model curiosity, not certainty. When possible, wonder aloud rather than correct ('I'm not sure, maybe we can think about that together'). This invites symbolic thinking and reduces black-and-white anxiety.
- Do not force exposures. Exposure work should always occur with therapeutic support once trust is built. Prematurely pushing the young person into feared situations can heighten persecution feelings.
- Contain rather than confront. A calm, containing response communicates that the fear can be survived and thought about. Confrontation or disbelief often increases defensive rituals.

Chapter 11

The Depressive Position in OCD

The radiators in the consulting room were only working intermittently, a fairly typical feature of a publicly funded service. Yet the dark winter afternoon, the condensation on the windows, and the low, bleak clouds seemed to match the mood of the young person sat in front of me. She was 14, her voice quiet but deliberate. 'I keep thinking I made my mum ill. She was sick last week and I know it was my fault because I wished she would leave me alone.' She looked down, ashamed. 'I didn't want it to happen. But I thought it. And then it did.'

She went on to describe how every small mistake in her rituals – missing a step when washing her hands, checking the door in the wrong order – felt like proof that she was careless and to blame. What stood out was not panic, nor silence, nor the atmosphere of catastrophe I had seen in other young people. Instead, there was a heaviness, a sadness that she could name and sit with, almost too much. The weight in the room was not of terror nor retreat but of grief and guilt. It genuinely felt like someone was sat in front of me highlighting all the mistakes they had ever made in their life.

Conceptual Overview: The Depressive Position in OCD

This is the depressive position. Often an unfortunate and misleading name, and misattributed to major depressive disorder or actual clinical depression, Melanie Klein (1935, 1940) described it as one of the earliest steps in emotional life: the realisation that the same person can be both loved and hated, good and bad, safe and frustrating. Crucially, this recognition is not only painful but also a developmental achievement. To bear ambivalence, to feel guilt, and to want to repair are signs of emotional growth and achievement. They open the door to empathy, mourning, and deeper relationships. Yet for adolescents with obsessive-compulsive disorder (OCD), this same achievement can feel unbearable. Intrusive thoughts arrive not just as unwanted intrusions, but as evidence of inner destructiveness. They say to themselves, 'The fact I thought it proves there is something bad inside me.' Their rituals are often less about avoiding catastrophe and more about putting something right, small acts of repair or penance to balance an inner sense of guilt.

DOI: 10.4324/9781003729716-11

Adolescence sharpens and intensifies the internal struggle of development. Margaret Rustin (1991) described this stage as a period of mourning: for the lost body of childhood, the idealised parents of latency, and the securities of a simpler self. I see this often in clinical practice. While some adolescents are eager to move forward without looking back, others feel weighed down by what is being left behind: the relative safety of latency, lighter responsibilities, and a sense of innocence that no longer fits. Compulsions within the depressive position can be understood as attempts to manage not only guilt but also the sadness that accompanies the transition from childhood to adolescence. It is important to keep in mind that adolescence typically unfolds after the initial transition to comprehensive school. The early years of settling in and adjusting to a new environment have passed, and the routine of school life becomes a constant theme. Timetables, homework, and pressure around GCSEs dominate daily experience. The novelty of the new setting fades, and, naturally, some may long to return to a simpler time to escape the mounting pressures.

Alongside this mourning comes the reality of a changing body. Alessandra Lemma (2010, 2014) has written about how adolescence can heighten self-consciousness and shame. As sexual feelings emerge, some young people feel exposed or even corrupted by them. In depressive-position OCD, intrusive thoughts about harm, sex, or morality are often felt not as random intrusions but as proof of inner badness. Compulsions then take on the quality of penance – attempts to prove worth or repair damage in the face of these new bodily and emotional realities.

When adolescents arrive in this position, the atmosphere is heavy rather than frantic. They do not wall themselves off, as in the claustrum, nor do they step back whenever feelings rise, as in the psychic retreat. They do not carry the atmosphere of imminent catastrophe that marks the paranoid–schizoid stance. Instead, they stay in contact, but burdened by guilt and sorrow. Their compulsions are not shields against danger but quiet acts of penance. This makes therapeutic work both challenging and full of possibility. Behavioural techniques such as exposure and response prevention can be effective here, but not simply because they confront the symptom. They work because they build on the adolescent's developmental achievement – their capacity to tolerate ambivalence and mourning helping them discover that guilt can be survived without endless rituals of repair.

Clinical Examples of the Depressive Position in OCD

Amelia

Amelia was 15 when she was referred after months of silent self-punishment. Her intrusive thoughts centred on harming her younger brother. She insisted she would never act on them, yet the guilt was so consuming that she rewrote her homework each evening until the pages were neat and flawless. If she smudged a word, she started again. If she thought an unkind thought toward her brother, she whispered a private apology under her breath.

What stood out was not panic or dread but a kind of weary sorrow. She told me, 'I know it's not real, but it still feels awful. I feel like a terrible person for even having that thought.' Her compulsions were less about preventing catastrophe than about making amends. The rituals carried the texture of penance. In the room I did not feel shut out, as in the claustrum, nor pressed into urgent reassurance, as in the paranoid schizoid position. Instead, I felt the weight of her guilt and the pull of her longing to put something right.

At times, she could sit with her feelings almost too much, looping back into shame. Yet this honesty also created space for therapeutic work. When I gently named that her rewriting might be her way of 'making up' for the thought, she nodded through tears. 'It's like I have to show I'm good,' she said. I found it exhausting just listening to the number of times she would repeat a trivial task and the energy she poured into it. The sadness was live, present, and reachable. It was here that exposure work found its foothold, not by dismissing the thought but by helping her test whether she could survive carrying it without endless repair.

Oliver

Oliver was 16 and described long rituals of checking his school bag late into the night. He was not afraid of burglars or accidents if something was forgotten. Instead, he explained, 'If I leave something out, it means I do not care enough, and then I am a bad son.' The link to his parents was immediate. He worried constantly that he had let them down, that his carelessness might show he did not value them.

The compulsions were not about averting danger but about repairing a bond. He would unpack and repack his bag until every item was present, as though the act of getting it right could erase the thought that he might disappoint. Sitting with him, I noticed the atmosphere was not anxious or closed, but heavy with self reproach. His checking had the quality of confession, repeated not to avoid catastrophe but to undo guilt.

When I asked what it felt like if he tried to stop the ritual, he replied, 'It would just prove I don't care. I couldn't bear that.' His words captured the essence of the depressive position: the fear that ambivalence means damage, and the desperate wish to repair through ritual. What struck me most was the cost. Oliver described spending hours repeating these tasks, and I felt drained just hearing the scale of effort. The exhaustion in the room was not only his but mine too, as though we were both carrying the burden of his endless attempts at repair.

Amelia and Oliver together illustrate the depressive position in OCD. Amelia shows how rituals can function as acts of penance, an attempt to prove goodness in the face of unbearable guilt. Oliver shows how checking can become a form of repair, a repeated effort to restore a bond that feels endangered. In both, the atmosphere was not one of panic, withdrawal, or sealed-off retreat, but of sadness and self-reproach. Their compulsions did not protect against catastrophe but carried the burden of guilt and the wish to make amends. What they share is the weight of mourning: a readiness to face the thought, but a conviction that it proves inner damage. It is this texture that marks the depressive position and that becomes evident in the consulting room, often as exhaustion for both adolescent and clinician.

The theory becomes clearest when seen in the room. The depressive position is not an abstract concept but a texture you can feel sitting opposite an adolescent: the weight of guilt, the pull toward penance, the sadness that does not drive them away but holds them in place. The following vignettes illustrate how this position takes shape in practice, showing how compulsions can function less as protection from catastrophe and more as acts of repair.

Sam

Sam was 16 and approached therapy as a project. He had read about OCD extensively online and quoted research papers with authority. 'I know it's just guilt,' he would say, 'a cognitive distortion.' Yet his tone carried a curious detachment, as if he were describing a patient other than himself. His knowledge seemed to provide temporary relief, a sense of control over feelings that otherwise felt overwhelming.

When he apologised for 'talking too much' or for 'not being a proper patient', I realised that intellect itself had become a ritual of repair – a way to cleanse guilt through explanation. Understanding offered momentary purity. But when emotion surfaced, the theory faltered, and the shame returned stronger. In session, I noticed my own admiration colliding with frustration. The words were right, but the feeling was missing.

Only when Sam admitted that reading about guilt 'made me feel cleaner' did the meaning of his compulsion come into view. His intellect was performing the same function as a washing ritual: an attempt to scrub away the stain of inner badness. For him, thinking was the compulsion, insight the detergent.

Clinical Transcripts: The Depressive Position

Amelia

Context: Amelia has described rewriting her homework repeatedly after an intrusive thought about her younger brother. The therapist explores the link between the thought, the guilt, and the compulsion.

THERAPIST: You told me you sometimes feel you have to start your work over. What makes you begin again?
AMELIA: Because if I leave it messy it proves I am careless.

(Annotation: Her words are not anxious or urgent but heavy with self-reproach. The ritual carries the meaning of penance, not protection.)

THERAPIST: So when you do rewrite it, how does that make you feel?
AMELIA: A little better, but not for long. The thought comes back.

(Annotation: Relief is temporary. The ritual is an attempt at repair but does not resolve the guilt. The sadness lingers in the room.)

THERAPIST: Do you ever think the ritual might be your way of making up for the thought?
AMELIA: (tears in her eyes): Yes. It is like I have to show I am good.

(Annotation: The depressive position is evident. She does not deny or ward off the feeling, she carries it, and the ritual becomes proof of goodness against feared destructiveness.)

THERAPIST: What happens if you do not rewrite it?
AMELIA: Then it means I do not care enough, and I could not live with that.

(Annotation: The catastrophe is not external. It is moral, centred on failing those she loves. The atmosphere is heavy rather than panicked.)

Oliver

Context: Oliver is describing his late-night checking of his school bag. The therapist explores the meaning behind the ritual.

THERAPIST: You said you often check your bag again and again before bed. What do you think will happen if you stop?
OLIVER: Nothing bad outside. It just means I do not care enough.

(Annotation: The focus is not on external catastrophe but on moral failure. The ritual functions as proof of care, not protection from danger.)

THERAPIST: So when everything is checked and in place, how does that leave you feeling?
OLIVER: Relieved for a while, but then I start again. I cannot risk it looking like I do not care.

(Annotation: Temporary relief mirrors Amelia's experience. The ritual repairs guilt only briefly before the burden returns.)

THERAPIST: What feels worst about not checking?
OLIVER: That it shows I am not a good son. That is harder than anything else.

(Annotation: The depressive position comes into view. The fear is of inner destructiveness and letting down loved figures, not external threat.)

THERAPIST: I wonder if the checking is your way of trying to put things right.
OLIVER: (sighs): Yes. Like proving I care. But it never feels enough.

(Annotation: The compulsion is experienced as a reparative act. The atmosphere in the room is one of sadness and exhaustion rather than dread.)

Commentary

The transcripts with Amelia and Oliver show how the depressive position takes shape in the consulting room. What stands out is not a fear of catastrophe in the outside world, nor the sealed-off silence of withdrawal, but a persistent moral weight. Both adolescents describe rituals that function as acts of repair, as if their motivations for carrying out the rituals are a way to fix something morally incomprehensible. Amelia rewrites her work to prove she is good. Oliver checks his bag to reassure himself he is a caring son. In each case, the ritual is not a shield against danger but a penance for guilt.

The atmosphere of these sessions was marked by heaviness and exhaustion. With Amelia, I felt the weight of her endless self-correction. With Oliver, I noticed how draining it was simply to hear the scale of his repeated checking. This countertransference mirrors the depressive stance itself: the sense that the adolescent is already carrying the guilt and that the clinician, too, is drawn into the labour of holding it.

Unlike the claustrum, where flatness prevails, or the paranoid–schizoid position, where fear presses urgently for reassurance, here the feelings are accessible and in most cases verbalised directly. The adolescent does not flee from sadness, they sit in it, sometimes for too long. This creates both a challenge and an opening. The challenge lies in the risk of being pulled into endless cycles of repair. The opening lies in the possibility of mourning, where guilt can be thought about rather than enacted.

How the Depressive Position Appears in the Room

These adolescents often arrive with striking emotional insight. In fact, I often find that when they arrive I am eager to work with them as, whilst they bring a degree of sadness, it feels manageable. They can talk about their inner life with honesty and depth, sometimes offering their own explanations before I can. Sometimes I wonder internally why they are even seeing me given the insight they appear to have, but I also wonder aloud why they are still struggling with their OCD despite having all this insight. They know that thoughts are not actions, yet that knowledge brings little, if any, comfort. Beneath the insight, lies an eroding self-condemnation.

Guilt and shame are not secondary discoveries in therapy. They are the starting point. The fear is not 'What if I do something bad?' but 'What if I already have?' Shame is rarely projected outward. It is carried inward, constant and critical.

Rituals often have a quiet, confessional quality. These young people do not accuse; they confess. They are not checking the locks, they are checking themselves, replaying conversations, dissecting motives, reviewing whether they were kind enough or careful enough. Perfectionism, over-apologising, and endless self-monitoring are common.

In the room, the atmosphere is heavy rather than frantic. I often find myself exhausted simply listening to the number of times a trivial task has been repeated. What lingers is not panic but sorrow. Even when an exposure succeeds, the adolescent may not feel relief. Instead they grieve, as if success itself proves that they are still unworthy.

What distinguishes the depressive position is that the adolescent does not flee feeling. They walk into it. They bring their guilt, their shame, and their sadness openly, and they ask, sometimes without words, whether they can still be good even with these thoughts.

Ambivalent Thinking

For many of the positions described up until now, difficulty holding ambivalence or tolerating uncertainty has been a central feature. The claustrum avoids conflict through enclosure, the retreat sidesteps feeling altogether, and the paranoid–schizoid collapses contradiction into stark opposites. However, in the depressive position, one characteristic is strikingly different. There is no difficulty in being able to hold ambivalence or carry two opposing views. The adolescent can recognise that love and hate, care and resentment, tenderness and aggression are directed toward the same person.

In the depressive position, the adolescent does not struggle to recognise ambivalence. On the contrary, they carry it almost too fully. A young person may speak with warmth about their mother and in the same breath describe an intrusive sexual or violent thought toward her. Unlike in the claustrum, they do not wall the thought off. Unlike in the paranoid–schizoid position, they do not collapse it into certainty of catastrophe. Instead, they confess it, again and again, as if the very recognition of mixed impulses proves inner corruption.

I have met many adolescents who feel compelled to tell their mother every sexual or violent thought that crosses their mind, urgently checking whether it is 'normal'. The ritual is not about preventing harm in the external world but about repairing an inner moral wound, reassuring themselves that they are still good, still loveable. In this sense, compulsions become acts of penance. As with Amelia, rewriting homework until perfect, rechecking a school bag late into the night, and whispering apologies under the breath are all variations on the same theme, attempts to repair what ambivalence has exposed.

As I outlined earlier, Klein (1935, 1940) described the depressive position as a developmental advance, allowing love and hate to be recognised as directed toward the same figure. In adolescent OCD, this same capacity is lived as a torment. The adolescent does not flee ambivalence. They sit in it, looping through guilt and confession, as though ordinary mixed feelings were evidence of inner destructiveness.

Internal Guilt

In the depressive position, guilt is directed inward. Unlike the paranoid–schizoid position, where blame is often projected outward onto objects or situations, here the adolescent carries the burden themselves. They see the thought as evidence of inner destructiveness rather than an external threat. The language is confessional rather than accusatory: 'I am careless,' 'It proves I am bad,' 'It means I do not care enough.'

This inward focus gives the rituals their reparative quality. Compulsions are not about neutralising danger in the outside world but about making amends for a perceived fault inside. The work of the clinician is often to notice how self-condemnation dominates the atmosphere, and how shame is carried with relentless weight.

Reflective Insight

These adolescents often speak with striking emotional honesty. They may offer their own explanations before the clinician asks, aware that the thought itself is irrational, yet unable to escape the guilt it provokes. They can articulate their inner world with unusual clarity, sometimes in ways that surprise their parents or teachers. Yet this insight does not bring relief. If anything, it deepens the self-criticism. Knowing that thoughts are not actions does not loosen the guilt; it confirms the sense that they should know better.

In the room, the reflective capacity is clear, but it does not bring lightness. The adolescent is not blind to their difficulty, they are caught in a loop of recognising it and condemning themselves for it.

Self-Punishing Rituals

Compulsions in the depressive position often take the form of penance. Rewriting, repeating, apologising, perfecting, or checking are not simply habits of control but acts of self-punishment. The ritual is carried out as if to repair damage already done or to prove moral worth in the face of inner doubt.

Clinically these rituals may appear endless. The adolescent explains that they must get it exactly right, not because catastrophe will strike but because failure would confirm they are careless or bad. The repetitive energy can be exhausting to hear about, let alone to live through. For the clinician, the countertransference often mirrors this fatigue, as though one has been drawn into the same weary cycle of reparation.

Mourning Process

Underlying the depressive stance is an awareness of loss. The adolescent often mourns an imagined purity or goodness they feel has already been spoiled by their intrusive thoughts. They grieve not for an external object but for a version of themselves they believe they have damaged. This sense of inner brokenness is what fuels both the sadness and the compulsion to repair.

In the consulting room, this mourning gives the atmosphere its weight. The clinician may feel as if sitting beside someone already in grief, except the lost object is the adolescent's own sense of worth. Work here often means holding steady enough for that mourning to be tolerated without being converted entirely into ritual.

Box 11.1 Recognising the Depressive Psychic Position

- Guilt and responsibility dominate. The young person feels personally accountable for harm, failure, or disappointment, even when evidence is thin.
- Compulsions serve to repair. Rituals are often driven by the wish to make amends or prevent loss rather than to ward off danger.
- Tone of sadness or apology. The atmosphere in the room feels heavy, remorseful, or quietly self-critical; reassurance rarely lifts it.
- Moral anxiety over contamination. The fear is less about dirt and more about moral stain or being 'a bad person'.
- Reluctance to burden others. The adolescent may under-report distress to protect family or therapist, creating a false sense of progress.
- Therapist countertransference of rescue. The clinician often feels pulled to comfort, rescue, or absolve, which can unintentionally maintain guilt.

Working Clinically with the Depressive Position

Working with adolescents in the depressive position requires a different stance from the clinician than in the other positions. Here the feelings are not avoided or projected but carried, often with openness that can be both moving and exhausting. The task is not to gain access to the emotional world but to tolerate the weight of guilt and the relentless drive to repair.

Holding the Atmosphere

Sessions are often marked by sorrow and heaviness. The adolescent may describe long, repetitive rituals of penance in such detail that even listening becomes tiring. This exhaustion is not incidental but part of the depressive atmosphere. It reflects the way guilt consumes energy and life feels like unending reparation. The clinician's role is to hold steady in this atmosphere without rushing to lighten it. Attempts at reassurance risk becoming another ritual. Instead, the work is to bear witness, to name the effort, and to show that the guilt can be shared in the room without collapsing into endless repair.

Witnessing and Containment

Because these adolescents already recognise their guilt, interpretation is less important than containment. They do not need help seeing what is wrong; they need help surviving the knowledge of it. The clinician offers containment by staying present, by naming what is being carried, and by showing that guilt and love can coexist. This witnessing stance can itself be reparative, demonstrating that the young person remains good and whole even when destructive thoughts are admitted.

Naming Repair without Collusion

Rituals in this position often carry the quality of penance. They are not just habits of control but acts of moral repair. The clinician can help by naming this function gently: 'It sounds like rewriting your work is your way of making up for the thought,' or 'I wonder if the checking is your way of showing you care.' Such remarks validate the underlying wish for repair whilst keeping the compulsive cycle visible. The aim is not to strip rituals away too quickly, which risks leaving the adolescent exposed, but to open the possibility of thinking about what the ritual is doing.

Finding the Foothold for ERP

Exposure and response prevention (ERP) can be especially effective in this position, but it must be carefully framed. The adolescent already knows the thought is irrational. The challenge is surviving the guilt rather than disproving the thought. ERP works when presented as an experiment in endurance: 'Let's see if you can carry the guilt without having to repair it right away.' When done with steadiness and care, ERP can show that guilt need not dictate endless ritual, that survival is possible without perpetual penance.

Balancing Depth with Behavioural Work

Work in the depressive position benefits from integrating behavioural and psychoanalytic approaches. ERP can create practical shifts, but its effectiveness depends on whether the adolescent feels that their guilt and grief are being recognised. When progress stalls, the question to ask is not simply 'What exposure is next?' but 'What emotion underlies the stuckness?' Often it is grief for a lost ideal of purity or goodness. Naming this grief can loosen the hold of rituals and open space for growth.

Supporting Mourning and Growth

At the core of the depressive position is mourning. The adolescent grieves an imagined goodness they believe to be spoiled by their thoughts. The clinician's role is to help them bear this mourning without collapsing into repair. This means showing that destructive and loving impulses can coexist, that the adolescent remains worthy even with both sides present. Bion (1962) described this as the slow work of thinking: feelings can be named, links made, truths spoken that once felt unbearable. When mourning is thought about rather than enacted, the possibility of growth becomes real.

The Therapist's Guilt and Hope

Working with guilt often stirs guilt. I have found that in the depressive position, the clinician's own capacity for self-reproach is tested. When an adolescent describes endless failures, I feel the reflex of my own wish to rescue or to make things better. In certain moments, I want to switch to a more solution-focused and problem-solving approach, perhaps slip into the role of a cheerleader. Sometimes, I sense my words as inadequate, my patience too short, my understanding too late. These are not signs of error but part of the shared depressive field. To hold hope in this atmosphere means accepting that repair will be slow and incomplete, and that we too must survive our limits. Again, something easier said then done.

The hope of the depressive position is not lightness but endurance – the slow discovery that guilt can coexist with love, and that care survives imperfection. When this becomes imaginable in the room, something fundamental shifts: mourning becomes creative rather than immobilising.

Guidance for Parents

(For clinicians to use when communicating with families.)

This section is not written as direct advice for parents but as language for clinicians to use when supporting families. The aim is to help parents understand the depressive position in a way that reduces shame, avoids jargon, and fosters steadiness at home.

Explaining the Role of Guilt

Clinicians can explain that some young people with OCD carry an unusually heavy burden of guilt. Parents may hear their child say 'I feel like a bad person' or 'It means I do not care enough.' The key message is that these statements reflect the depressive position: the child is not avoiding feelings but is weighed down by them. Helping parents see this reframes the behaviour not as defiance or drama but as the adolescent struggling with overwhelming self-condemnation.

Understanding Rituals as Repair

Families often wonder why their child keeps repeating trivial tasks or apologising endlessly. Clinicians can frame these rituals as attempts to make up for guilt rather than as meaningless habits. Explaining that the child is not preventing danger but trying to repair an imagined wrong helps parents respond with compassion rather than frustration. They can then encourage small steps away from ritual without demanding that the guilt vanish overnight.

How to Respond at Home

Parents may feel torn between wanting to reassure and fearing that reassurance fuels the OCD. Clinicians can suggest simple language that validates effort without colluding with the compulsion. For example: 'I can see you feel bad and are trying hard to make it right,' instead of repeating reassurance that nothing bad happened. This approach acknowledges the guilt while gently reducing the cycle of repair.

Creating a Steady Atmosphere

Because the depressive position is marked by heaviness and mourning, home life can easily feel drained. Clinicians can help parents by naming this atmosphere and encouraging steadiness rather than constant attempts to cheer the adolescent up. Consistency, patience, and recognition of effort are more helpful than repeated reassurances or dramatic interventions. The task is not to erase guilt but to support the adolescent in carrying it until they can find new ways of living with it.

Parents, too, can be drawn into the depressive atmosphere. They may feel guilty for not noticing sooner or for having been frustrated in the past. The clinician's role is to model forgiveness here as well: to show that guilt in families can be thought about rather than expiated through overprotection. When parents can bear their own guilt without passing it back to the child, the household atmosphere lightens for everyone.

Summary and Clinical Take Home

The depressive position is marked not by avoidance of feeling but by the painful capacity to carry ambivalence, guilt, and sadness. Adolescents in this stance often show unusual emotional honesty and reflective insight, yet their rituals reveal a cycle of self-punishment and repair. Unlike the claustrum or retreat, they do not flee from their feelings; unlike the paranoid schizoid position, they do not project catastrophe outward. They sit with guilt, sometimes too much, and try to undo it through ritual.

For clinicians, the atmosphere in the room is heavy, often exhausting. The countertransference mirrors the adolescent's labour, as though both are caught in the weight of mourning. ERP can find its strongest foothold here, provided it is paced carefully and framed as an experiment in surviving guilt without endless repair. Symbolic work and behavioural work can meet most fully in this position, where mourning becomes thinkable and growth possible.

> **Box 11.2 ERP and the Depressive Position: When to Pause and When to Proceed**
>
> - Proceed when guilt can be thought about, not obeyed. Begin ERP once the young person can recognise guilt as a feeling, not a fact demanding punishment.
> - Pause if exposures turn into self-punishment. When tasks are used to atone or prove goodness, the work reinforces depression rather than reducing obsession.
> - Proceed with gentle collaboration. Frame ERP as shared inquiry: 'Let's see what happens if we test that belief together.'
> - Pause when affect becomes flat or despairing. If hope collapses, containment must come before exposure; otherwise ERP becomes another proof of failure.
> - Proceed when meaning is integrated. When the adolescent can link the ritual to themes of loss or responsibility, exposure can help test those links safely.
> - Pause if family pressure dominates. ERP should not serve others' relief from guilt; it must emerge from the young person's own readiness.

> **Box 11.3 Clinician's Guidance to Parents**
>
> - Recognise guilt as emotion, not truth. Help parents understand that apologies or self-criticism signal distress, not moral failing.
> - Respond with steadiness, not reassurance. 'You haven't done anything wrong' may not reach them; calm presence is more containing.
> - Notice signs of hidden despair. Withdrawn quietness or apparent compliance can mask hopelessness that needs gentle inquiry.
> - Encourage balanced responsibility. Support the adolescent to take age-appropriate ownership without collapsing into blame or avoidance.
> - Avoid over-rescuing. Parents' instinct to comfort or fix can inadvertently confirm the young person's sense of badness or incompetence.
> - Model forgiveness and perspective. Naming that everyone makes mistakes helps re-establish a realistic, human moral frame.
> - Celebrate repair attempts, not perfection. Small moments of courage, honesty, or relational repair are signs of movement out of depressive guilt.

References

Bion, W. R. (1962). *Learning from experience.* London: Heinemann.

Klein, M. (1935). A contribution to the psychogenesis of manic-depressive states. *The International Journal of Psychoanalysis*, 16, 145–174.

Klein, M. (1940). Mourning and its relation to manic-depressive states. *The International Journal of Psychoanalysis*, 21, 125–153.

Lemma, A. (2010). *Under the skin: A psychoanalytic study of body modification.* London and New York: Routledge.

Lemma, A. (2014). *Minding the body: The body in psychoanalysis and beyond.* London and New York: Routledge.

Rustin, M. (1991). *The good society and the inner world: Psychoanalytic, social, and political perspectives.* London: Verso.

Chapter 12

Measuring the Invisible – Integrating Reflection and Evidence

One of the greatest challenges in researching internal processes is how to measure them. We can count compulsions, administer psychometric scales, or even generate transcripts from audio recordings, yet something vital slips through. The clinical atmosphere, the subtle shifts, the undercurrents, the unspoken resonance resists capture. Our instruments record the surface but miss the psychic process itself.

Freud's 'Rat Man' case (1955) showed how meticulous description could illuminate inner life, but such accounts resisted generalisation. Later, tools like the Children's Yale–Brown Obsessive Compulsive Scale (CY-BOCS; Skahill et al., 1997) brought standardisation and allowed data to be collated across samples. Behavioural indices further refined our ability to judge improvement. Yet, even with these advances, what remains unmeasured is the adolescent's stance toward their thoughts, the psychic position from which they suffer.

Throughout this book I have argued that the four positions – claustrum, paranoid-schizoid, psychic retreat, and depressive – offer a more precise lens on intrusive thoughts and subsequent compulsions. But positions cannot be reduced to numbers. They are clinical concepts, honed over decades of psychoanalytic work and sharpened in the consulting room through supervision, reflection, and note-taking. Attempts to turn them into psychometric tools are premature. What proves more useful now is a reflective framework, one that can be taught in supervision and applied flexibly.

When I began introducing these positions to trainees and colleagues from different disciplines – psychiatry, psychology, nursing, counselling – I quickly realised that what mattered most was not a set of diagnostic items but a shared way of noticing. In supervision, I would encourage them to set aside the checklist for a moment and ask instead: what does it feel like to sit with this adolescent? Is the atmosphere thick with absence, as if contact is sealed off? Does the young person appear fluent and articulate until emotion rises, at which point their symptoms flare? Is the world divided into black and white, with no room for ambiguity? Or is there a tentative capacity for ambivalence, guilt, and repair?

DOI: 10.4324/9781003729716-12

These impressions are not 'soft data'. They are the clinician's primary instrument. When gathered systematically through reflection, supervision, and careful note-taking, they begin to form a pattern that can orient us to the psychic position. This reflective measure does not produce a numerical score but it does generate a working hypothesis, one that is clinically useful. In particular, it can help decide whether exposure and response prevention (ERP) is appropriate. For example, a young person in a depressive position may be able to tolerate graded ERP, whereas one locked in a claustrum may experience such work as unbearable intrusion.

I have found it most useful to frame this not as a separate assessment tool but as a scaffold for supervision. After presenting a case, trainees are invited to map their experience of the adolescent against the four positions. They consider their countertransference, the quality of the adolescent's speech, the pattern of symptom fluctuation, and the way meaning is either avoided or allowed. Over time, these reflections sharpen into a clinical sensibility that complements, rather than replaces, formal measures such as the CY-BOCS.

What emerges is a form of measurement that honours both science and atmosphere. It does not claim to be a new psychometric scale that will come, perhaps, in the future, with careful piloting and validation. For now, it is a structured way of holding the invisible in view, of giving language to what clinicians already feel but often struggle to describe.

Supervision Example – One Step Forward, Two Steps Back

I recall supervising a trainee who was working with a 14-year-old girl with severe obsessive-compulsive disorder (OCD), confirmed by a high score on the CY-BOCS. On the surface, everything appeared to be going well. The trainee described a good therapeutic alliance, weekly sessions, and supportive parents. Some weeks, the young person made dramatic gains: she reported few intrusive thoughts, resisted compulsions, and described being able to 'ignore the OCD'. On other weeks she felt overwhelmed. Her compulsions escalated, the intrusive thoughts became unbearable, and the trainee felt bewildered by the inconsistency.

The trainee had tried behavioural analysis, but the setbacks followed no obvious pattern. Reviewing an audio transcript together, the missing thread emerged, whenever disappointment or rejection was touched conflict with a teacher, tension with her mother, silence from a friend, her intrusive thoughts intensified sharply.

This discovery reframed the case. On paper, she looked like a straightforward candidate for ERP: motivated, engaged, with a good therapeutic alliance and committed parents. Yet ERP kept faltering. When we considered the possibility of a psychic retreat position, the pieces began to fall into place. Her OCD was not simply fluctuating with external stress; it was stepping in to manage the intolerable feelings of rejection that surfaced in relationships.

The supervision process then shifted. The trainee began to help her notice these links gently, without rushing into exposure tasks. Sessions became rockier. She missed appointments, pulled back at times, and the smooth trajectory of earlier work broke down. Gradually, however, she began to articulate the feelings that triggered her symptoms. She described how a friend's silence on text, especially when she saw that same friend active on Snapchat, felt like rejection of the harshest kind. In her world, the logic was simple: if her friend could post, she could reply. Not replying meant she was being dismissed. Each time this feeling arose, her hand-washing rituals escalated.

By making this link explicit, the clinician and young person could begin to sit with the pain of rejection rather than letting the compulsions carry it. As this process unfolded, her OCD symptoms reduced. What had looked like inconsistency was in fact coherence. Her intrusive thoughts were serving as a retreat from unbearable affect. Once this was recognised, the work could deepen, and ERP became possible again, although at a different pace.

Commentary

This case illustrates how supervision can function as a reflective measure in its own right. Standard tools such as the CY-BOCS confirmed severity, but they could not explain why progress was uneven. It was only through reviewing transcripts and inviting the trainee to notice his own feelings in the room that the pattern became visible. The adolescent's symptoms were not random fluctuations. They escalated whenever disappointment or rejection entered the frame.

The reflective measure works by combining three sources of information: the young person's narrative, the atmosphere in the consulting room, and the clinician's countertransference. When these are examined together, the underlying position often reveals itself. In this case, the pattern of sudden withdrawal and symptom flare in the face of rejection pointed clearly to the psychic retreat.

For clinicians, the teaching point is twofold. First, positions cannot be captured by behavioural analysis alone. They show themselves in the relational field, not only in symptom charts. Second, recognising the position allows treatment to be paced more realistically. ERP was not abandoned, but it was reshaped to include time for noticing and bearing feelings of rejection. This shift in stance allowed progress that behavioural techniques on their own had not achieved.

ERP Collapses in the Claustrum

I once supervised a counselling student working with a 15-year-old girl whose intrusive thoughts focused on her stepfather. Sessions were marked by silence and an airless quality. The trainee described feeling drained, as if nothing could move. Out of frustration, he introduced ERP in a blunt, either–or frame. The result was a hostile encounter and abrupt dropout.

In supervision we reframed this as a claustral state. The suffocation he felt was not resistance but evidence of psychic retreat, where compulsions function as glue holding the self together. In this position, ERP cannot be forced; it is experienced as intrusion and risks collapse. The lesson was stark: what appears as hostility or indifference may in fact be survival. The task is not to insist on exposure but to recognise the claustral atmosphere and pace the work so the fragile structure is not threatened.

Cases like this bring the dilemma into sharp relief. On paper, her severity could have been indexed neatly with the CY-BOCS, and progress could have been tracked session by session. Yet none of those numbers would have explained why ERP collapsed so abruptly, or why the atmosphere in the room felt so airless. It is here that the limits of psychometric measurement become most apparent and it is also here that I anticipate the strongest criticism of the framework I am proposing.

Anticipating the Evidence-based Critique

In contemporary services shaped by NICE guidelines, CY-BOCS scores, and throughput targets, it is inevitable that a framework such as this will be questioned. Where is the evidence base? How can it be measured? These are fair questions, and psychometric tools do have their place. They provide consistency, they allow outcomes to be compared across studies, and they reassure commissioners that young people are improving, and the interventions are being in a competent manner.

But in child and adolescent services, the pressure to demonstrate progress quickly can narrow our attention. Symptoms are indexed, sessions are counted, and outcomes are defined in terms of diagnostic criteria. This can be helpful, as I acknowledged in Chapter 2, but it also risks flattening the uniqueness of the individual into a score. When the clinical presentation is reduced to a standardised assessment, we lose sight of the texture of the therapeutic encounter such as the atmosphere, the countertransference, the lived stance of the adolescent toward their intrusive thoughts.

I do not dismiss psychometric measures. They anchor research and guide best practice. But I am equally aware that this framework will be criticised for lacking them. There are, as yet, no validated questionnaires that can locate a young person in a claustrum or a psychic retreat. What we have instead is practice-based evidence, the disciplined noticing of what it feels like to sit with the adolescent, how symptoms flare when feelings rise, and how the position itself organises the clinical encounter. To my mind, that is evidence of a different but no less necessary kind.

Reflective Measures as Clinical Instruments

What I am setting out here is not another checklist and it is not a new scale. It is a way of paying attention that is already part of clinical work, but needs to be made more deliberate. In supervision I encourage trainees to notice their countertransference, to listen to the quality of the young person's speech, and to think about how symptoms rise and fall across sessions. These are not numbers, but they do form data of a kind. They give us orientation.

I am not suggesting we throw away the measures we already have. The CY-BOCS and other scales are important and they keep us accountable. But they cannot tell us about the stance the adolescent takes toward their OCD. That is what matters most to me. I want to know what their relationship to the compulsion is, how it sits in the room, and what it does to the atmosphere between us. If we can bring that alive, the young person can begin to test whether they still need to cling to the ritual in the way they do.

A lot of this sounds simple, but it is easily missed. We get busy planning interventions, thinking about behavioural experiments, involving families, and working through protocols. All of that matters. Yet, in the middle of it, small things can slip past us. The way a sentence shuts down just as feeling comes close. The sense of airlessness or stuckness in the room. Our own pull to rescue or to push harder. These are not minor details. They are the very material that tells us what position we are in.

It also needs patience. The first few sessions often reflect ordinary adolescent process: nerves, anger at being sent, boredom, or guardedness. That does not mean the young person is in a claustrum or a psychic retreat. We have to give time for the clinical texture to unfold. In my experience it is only after several sessions, when we know something of their daily life and how OCD interferes, that the relationship with the symptom becomes clearer.

When this understanding is there, ERP can be approached more safely. I have found that once I share a sense of the position with the adolescent, without jargon and in simple words, they often have more confidence in resisting compulsions. It does not always need a heavy-handed exposure task. Sometimes the urgency softens just by knowing what the symptom has been doing for them. If we rush ERP because we are counting sessions, the risk of collapse is much higher.

So the point I am making is that we need both. We need the established evidence base and the reflective, practice-based evidence that comes from atmosphere, stance, and countertransference. Only when they are held together can we pace treatment well enough to avoid harm and to give the young person a chance to work with, rather than against, their own mind.

The Horizon of Operationalisation

Although I have argued throughout that these positions are hard to quantify, I do not want to say they should never be operationalised. I hope that one day they might be, though I think any measure would always be incomplete. Even with audio or video recordings we cannot fully capture countertransference or the intersubjective feel of a session. Something will always exceed the categories.

What does seem possible, though, is to begin with transcripts. If transcripts were annotated, not only with the adolescent's words but also with the clinician's countertransference at key moments, I believe patterns would emerge. This would rely on clinicians being self-reflective, ideally supported by personal therapy or other reflective practice, so they could name and separate their own feelings. If such transcripts were coded over time, I suspect we would start to see recognisable markers of position.

For example, in the claustrum there is often a closed-down quality to language, short or snappy sentences, a sense of being trapped. There is usually little reference to external threat. Clinicians consistently report feeling stuck or suffocated in these sessions. These are not abstract descriptors. They are reliable clinical experiences that point to the claustral position. If we could find a way to capture these patterns systematically, it would give researchers and commissioners a new language for what is already being lived in the room.

I think this could be an important step. It might encourage services not to rush ERP within a set number of sessions, but to pace the work according to stance. Over time, with evolution of clinical practice, we might arrive at measures of position that, while never complete, help us predict treatment readiness. That in turn could improve the effectiveness of ERP, reduce relapse, and improve quality of life for adolescents with OCD.

For me, this is the direction the field needs to move in. We cannot keep circling back to the same strategies, challenging beliefs, persuasion, motivational interviewing as if conviction alone could make exposures possible. No matter how creative we are, ERP fails when the adolescent's relationship to their OCD has not been understood. Until that is the starting point, we will remain at an impasse. And even if progress is made, relapse is likely when the deeper stance has not shifted.

Holding the Invisible in View

The task, then, is not to reject measurement but to widen it. Numbers will always be necessary, but they are not sufficient. To honour what happens in the consulting room, we must also measure atmosphere, stance, and survival – however imprecise those measures may seem. In doing so, we keep the invisible in view, resisting the temptation to treat what cannot be quantified as if it does not exist.

What I have tried to do in this book is show that the framework is not an attack on cognitive behavioural therapy (CBT), nor a dismissal of ERP, nor a claim that research evidence is somehow mistaken. Some colleagues do take that hard line, but I do not. The empirical findings remain essential. Numerical data, carefully collected, tell us a great deal about mechanisms that maintain obsessive-compulsive symptoms, especially in adolescence. That body of work is fruitful and deserves respect.

But alongside it, we must remember what is harder to capture: the positions, the atmosphere, the relationship the young person has with their OCD. These are not yet open to quantification, except perhaps in detailed case studies or in annotated transcripts that combine the adolescent's words with the clinician's countertransference. They are part of the picture, even if they do not fit easily into a research protocol.

My own stance is integrationist. As a clinical psychologist, I am trained to think across modalities, and I see value in holding quantitative and qualitative approaches together. We do not need to discard CBT, or behavioural science, or the vast work of cognitive researchers. But nor should we ignore the contributions of psychoanalytic theory, which has been observing and describing these processes for nearly a century. Integration here does not mean throwing ideas together at random, or chasing novelty. It means working carefully, with respect for both traditions, and extracting what still shines from older papers while setting it beside contemporary research.

This is, in part, why the book came into being. Immersing myself in the older psychoanalytic literature, while reflecting on my own practice and supervision, I found an intuitive thread that seemed to demand words on paper. My hope is that others who share a respect for both effective psychological intervention and the theoretical work of those who came before us will recognise that thread too. At its best, it can help us hold a light in the otherwise dark and repetitive loops of obsession and compulsion.

In the end, what I am calling for is not a new scale but a way of keeping the invisible in view. Numbers will continue to matter, but so will atmosphere, stance, and the weight of what it feels like to sit in the room with a young person. If this book has offered anything, I hope it is a reminder that our measures must be broad enough to include both: the scores that reassure us we are making progress, and the lived experience that tells us whether that progress will last. The next chapter steps outside the language of measures altogether, and turns instead to reflection on what it means to sit with obsession, to stay with compulsion, and to listen for meaning where numbers fall silent.

References

Freud, S. (1955). *Notes upon a case of obsessional neurosis* [*'Rat Man' case*]. In J. Strachey (Ed. & Trans.), *The standard edition of the complete psychological works of Sigmund Freud* (Vol. 10, pp. 153–318). London: Hogarth Press. (Original work published 1909.)

Scahill, L., Riddle, M. A., McSwiggin-Hardin, M., Ort, S. I., King, R. A., & Goodman, W. K., Leckman, J. F. (1997). Children's Yale–Brown Obsessive Compulsive Scale: Reliability and validity. *Journal of the American Academy of Child & Adolescent Psychiatry*, 36 (6), 844–852. doi:10.1097/00004583-199706000-00023.

Chapter 13

Closing Reflections

What I have set out in this book is not a new method, and certainly not a rival to cognitive behavioural therapy (CBT) or exposure and response prevention (ERP). It is simply a way of working that keeps the relationship at the centre and treats obsessive-compulsive disorder (OCD) as more than a checklist of symptoms. Colleagues sometimes describe it as a kind of 'pre-ERP' approach. That may simplify the idea, but there is some truth in it: the ground has to be prepared before the harder exposures can take root.

For me, what matters most is not the content of the obsessions or compulsions, but the relationship the adolescent has with them. By this, I do not mean only whether they fear their symptoms, find comfort in them, or secretly value them. Those are surface attitudes. Beneath them lies something deeper: the psychic position from which the adolescent meets their OCD. That stance, the way the disorder is lived in the inner world, shapes everything.

I have tried to show that therapy is not about cleverness or clever techniques. It is about sitting with a young person in their particular stance, sometimes in silence, sometimes amid urgency, sometimes with tears, and recognising what the OCD means for them at that moment. When we can do that, techniques like ERP have a chance to work with, rather than against, the young person's psychic reality.

As can be seen throughout numerous examples in this book, on the surface, young people may have looked similar. The themes repeated: contamination, harm, sexuality, morality. Yet, underneath, their positions were different. Some were shut down, unreachable. Some were flooded with guilt. Some retreated into rituals as if they were a refuge. Some were open and desperate to speak. The task was not to apply a fixed set of techniques, but to recognise the position and meet it with the right stance.

Everything we know about therapy points to the same truth: success depends on the relationship. And that relationship is more than rapport or trust-building. It is about finding a footing together, a shared place to stand in the work. When I could name and recognise the dominant position with a young person, and respond to it directly, things often began to shift. Not instantly and not dramatically, but slowly, as though the atmosphere in the

DOI: 10.4324/9781003729716-13

room became lighter. The young person sensed I was not pushing them into tasks they were not ready for, and that made space for curiosity, for wondering, and for hope.

This did not mean that ERP was set aside, or that exposure could be avoided altogether. At some stage, most adolescents with OCD needed to confront the things they feared and resist the rituals that held them captive. What changed was the pacing. It was not about spending weeks on trust-building exercises as a prelude. It was about understanding the structure of their mind and how they were relating to their OCD. When ERP came, it came in a way that felt possible, not forced.

Too often, I have seen young people disengage when ERP was introduced too early, or pressed without attention to psychic position. Sometimes it worked beautifully with little preparation; sometimes it caused harm. This was not a question of skill or effort, but of readiness. If a young person was walled off in the claustrum, ERP could feel like a violation. If they were in a more depressive position, it could be a vital step forward. Knowing the difference was what mattered.

Patience was essential. This was what Bion (1970) called negative capability, borrowing from the poet Keats: the capacity to sit with uncertainty and not rush to solutions. Clinicians struggled with this, myself included. We wanted change, and we wanted to offer reassurance. But reassurance itself could become part of the ritual, and rushing too quickly could close things down. The discipline was to wait, to bear the discomfort of not knowing, and to allow something real to emerge.

This model was not a cure-all. It was not the only way of working with OCD. I saw adolescents improve through psychoeducation, parent work, and ERP alone. I saw others respond best to ideas drawn from acceptance and commitment therapy. The point was never to privilege one approach over another, but to hold to the principle of what works for whom.

What I came to believe was that when we could understand the architecture of a young mind, especially during the turbulence of adolescence, we could help more effectively. These were years when the psyche was already chaotic, when identity, sexuality, morality, and belonging were all in flux. It was no surprise that intrusive thoughts, with their intensity and strangeness, so often appeared at this stage.

A question I was often asked was whether young people stayed in one position, or moved between them. My answer was that there was nearly always a dominant position, at least in the early and middle stages of therapy. But positions were not fixed. Adolescents could move between paranoid–schizoid and depressive states, sometimes even in the space of a session. They could jump back into defended retreats when things felt overwhelming. It was not linear, and it was not predictable, but it was recognisable.

In the room, you felt it. Words that landed and went nowhere. The sense of being shut out. The feeling of being tested or persecuted. Or, at the other end, the weight of guilt and honesty that filled the atmosphere. These were not minor shifts in mood but signals of psychic position. Once I learned to trust what they stirred in me, they became a guide.

Challenges and Extensions

This framework did not downplay compulsions or ignore the role of ERP. Rituals were central to the lived reality of OCD, often giving the clearest clues to the underlying position: repeated washing as moral cleansing, checking as a guard against psychic fragmentation, confession as penance. Recognising the position helped explain why compulsions took the form they did, and when it was safe to invite the adolescent to resist them.

Nor was this model intended to delay ERP indefinitely. Exposure and response prevention remains the evidence-based foundation of treatment, but its timing and framing depend on whether the young person can bear the encounter. The positions orient us to readiness, not avoidance.

I also acknowledged that identifying a dominant position is never a precise science. At best, it is a clinical judgement tested and retested in the ongoing relationship. Positions shift, sometimes quickly, and what matters is that we remain flexible enough to notice and respond.

A final question remains: do these four positions apply only to obsessive–compulsive disorder, or might they extend more widely across adolescent psychopathology? My own experience leads me to a cautious answer.

It is true that elements of these psychic stances can be recognised in many presentations. Anorexia nervosa, for example, is perhaps one of the clearest conditions in which a claustrum-like position becomes visible. I have met young people who are emaciated, tube-fed, and medically at risk, yet who continue to insist they are overweight and must not eat. The fortress of anorexia functions not unlike the claustrum: a rigid, isolating psychic enclosure that protects against unbearable feelings at devastating personal cost. Similarly, health anxiety often has a paranoid–schizoid quality, where catastrophe is constantly imagined as imminent and external. Depressive disorders, by contrast, are suffused with the direct burden of loss and guilt. These resonances are real, and they suggest that the four positions may indeed provide a broader language for adolescent suffering.

And yet OCD remains distinct. At its core, every compulsion is tethered to an intrusive thought. It is these thoughts that crystallise the positions: walled-off in the claustrum, besieged in the paranoid–schizoid, hidden within retreat, or fully exposed in depressive guilt. No other disorder reveals such visible movement between positions, moment to moment, session to session. This is why OCD provides the clearest window through which to observe them.

We must also recognise the turbulence of adolescence itself. Puberty, sexuality, identity, and moral awakening all pressurise the adolescent mind. These forces shape not only the content of intrusive thoughts but the position the young person adopts toward them. In this sense, adolescence acts as the accelerant: it explains why OCD in young people so often carries the fluidity and intensity that bring the four positions into focus.

For these reasons, I present the model first and foremost as a framework for OCD in adolescence, while remaining open to its wider application. Future research may extend its use across other disorders, but my hope here is more modest: to sharpen our ear for the psychic positions that organise intrusive thoughts, and to offer clinicians a way of working that is both practical and deeply attuned. To recognise position is not to pathologise adolescence, but to give language to its turbulence, and in doing so to offer adolescents with OCD a clearer, more compassionate path through it.

If the book has one message, it is that OCD in adolescence is not only a set of symptoms to be managed but a relationship to be understood. When clinicians can recognise the psychic positions that shape this relationship, the work becomes not just possible, but humane.

Reference

Bion, W. R. (1970). *Attention and interpretation: A scientific approach to insight in psycho-analysis and groups.* London: Tavistock Publications.

Index

For Product Safety Concerns and Information please contact our EU
representative GPSR@taylorandfrancis.com
Taylor & Francis Verlag GmbH, Kaufingerstraße 24, 80331 München, Germany